# Introduction to
# NURSING
# RESEARCH

# Introduction to
# NURSING
# RESEARCH

## Developing Research Awareness

**Andrée le May**  BSc (Hons) RGN PhD PGCE(A) FRSPH
Formerly Professor of Nursing, School of Health
Sciences, University of Southampton, UK

**Susan Holmes**  BSc (Hons) PhD SRN FRSPH CMS
Director of Research and Development (Health and
Social Care) and Professor of Nursing, Canterbury Christ
Church University, UK

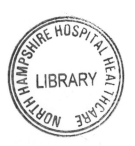
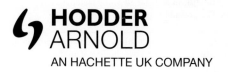
HODDER
ARNOLD
AN HACHETTE UK COMPANY

First published in Great Britain in 2012 by
Hodder Arnold, an imprint of Hodder Education, Hodder and Stoughton Ltd, a division of Hachette UK
338 Euston Road, London NW1 3BH

http://www.hodderarnold.com

© 2012 Andrée le May and Susan Holmes

Hachette UK's policy is to use papers that are natural, renewable and recyclable products and made from wood grown in sustainable forests. The logging and manufacturing processes are expected to conform to the environmental regulations of the country of origin.

Whilst the advice and information in this book are believed to be true and accurate at the date of going to press, neither the author[s] nor the publisher can accept any legal responsibility or liability for any errors or omissions that may be made. In particular, (but without limiting the generality of the preceding disclaimer) every effort has been made to check drug dosages; however, it is still possible that errors have been missed. Furthermore, dosage schedules are constantly being revised and new side-effects recognized. For these reasons the reader is strongly urged to consult the drug companies' printed instructions, and their websites, before administering any of the drugs recommended in this book.

British Library Cataloguing in Publication Data
A catalogue record for this book is available from the British Library

Library of Congress Cataloging-in-Publication Data
A catalog record for this book is available from the Library of Congress

ISBN-13    978-1-444-11990-9

1 2 3 4 5 6 7 8 9 10

Commissioning Editor:        Naomi Wilkinson
Project Editor:              Mischa Barrett
Production Controller:       Francesca Wardell
Cover Design:               Lynda King
Indexer:                    Laurence Errington

Cover image © Anna Tyukhmeneva


Typeset in Minion Regular 10 pts by Datapage (India) Pvt. Ltd.
Printed and bound in Spain by Graphycems

What do you think about this book? Or any other Hodder Arnold title?
Please visit our website: www.hodderarnold.com

# Contents

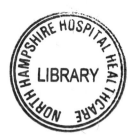

# Abbreviations

| | |
|---|---|
| CASP | Critical Appraisal Skills Programme |
| CINAHL | Cumulative Index of Nursing and Allied Health Literature |
| CLAHRC | Collaborations for Leadership in Applied Health Research and Care |
| CQC | Care Quality Commission |
| DARE | Database of Abstracts of Reviews of Effects |
| DH | Department of Health |
| DHSS | Department of Health and Social Security |
| EBP | evidence-based practice |
| HQIP | Healthcare Quality Improvement Partnership |
| HRQL | health-related quality of life |
| ICU | intensive care unit |
| IRAS | Integrated Research Application System |
| JBI | Joanna Briggs Institute |
| KTA | Knowledge-to-Action |
| LREC | Local Research Ethics Committee |
| MREC | Multicentre Research Ethics Committee |
| NHS | National Health Service |
| NICE | National Institute for Health and Clinical Excellence |
| NIHR | National Institute for Health Research |
| NIHR-SDO | National Institute for Health Research Service Delivery and Organisation programme |
| NMC | Nursing and Midwifery Council |
| NMEIT | No Material Ethical Issues Tool |
| NPSA | National Patient Safety Agency |
| NRES | National Research Ethics Service |
| NSF | National Service Framework |
| OMRU | Ottawa Model of Research Use |
| ONS | Office for National Statistics |
| PARiHS | Promoting Action on Research Implementation in Health Services |
| PHR | (The) Public Health Research programme |
| PIS | Participant Information Sheet |
| PR | proportionate review |
| PRSC | Proportionate Review Subcommittee |
| QI | quality improvement |
| QL | quality of life |
| R&D | research and development |

| | |
|---|---|
| RCN | Royal College of Nursing |
| RCT | randomized controlled trial |
| REC | Research Ethics Committee |
| RGF | Research Governance Framework |
| SCREC | Social Care Research Ethics Committee |

# Introduction

As students of nursing you may be wondering why you need a book about research or research awareness – what on earth has this got to do with my desire to be a nurse, to care for people? You may also question why or how research will make you a better nurse or enhance your practice. The answer is quite simple: it has everything to do with nursing! Research links theory with education and practice, enabling you to 'grow' your knowledge, enhance your critical thinking abilities and, increasingly, make better clinical judgements and informed decisions to the ultimate benefit of your patients.

The healthcare environment is constantly changing and the demands on nurses are significant as they are challenged to constantly improve the care they provide. This can't be achieved without awareness and knowledge of research if we are to gain the evidence needed to underpin effective care. Nurses must not only keep themselves up to date but also develop innovative approaches to 'old' problems and make a real difference to the patients in their care. This can be achieved only by developing a body of knowledge to underpin nursing practice – this is the role of research. Indeed, having a unique and specialized body of scientifically derived knowledge is one of the hallmarks of our profession and enhances our accountability to our patients. Nurses all over the world are working to expand our knowledge and enhance our practice; we must attempt to keep up with them. Knowledge that remains in the journals does little to improve patient care.

Understanding and using research in practice thus helps us to transform the knowledge research generates into practical and useful interventions or approaches to care and, through this, to make our practice truly evidence-based. Today, more than ever before, we are required to be accountable for the quality of the care we deliver and our Code of Professional Conduct requires that we are always able to justify our decisions. Research helps us to do this by validating nursing interventions or developing new approaches to care. In other words, research helps nursing to continue to advance.

We have designed this book to tempt you to explore the exciting and satisfying world of nursing research. Not all practitioners are expected to conduct research, though they are expected to be aware of and able to implement research findings, to be consumers of research; all nurses must be able to evaluate and use new knowledge in practice.

Why is research exciting – or satisfying? Well, think about the 'whodunnit' – working out who committed a murder, who stole the money or committed the crime – this is not dissimilar to the process(es) of nursing research. In both cases, we identify the question(s), search for clues using a variety of appropriate methods and put them together to solve the crime or problem. Finding the answer – and knowing you worked it out – provides the excitement of research; the satisfaction comes from disseminating the results to allow others to learn from its findings, making sure research is not only an academic endeavour but one that allows lessons to be learned and care to be improved. Knowing that your work has stimulated change is immensely gratifying.

If you're looking for a detailed text to tell you *how* to do research, this book provides only the basic ideas and an overview of its techniques; but if you're seeking a guide to its principles and the value of different types of research to nursing, we hope you will find it here. This is a book *about* research, introducing its ideas and concepts, establishing its basic principles and helping to guide your future in research whether as a user/consumer of its findings or a provider of its results.

In the following chapters we take you on a journey through the world of research. We start by considering how using research advances nursing care, then move on to focus on three examples of research-based practice, key elements that we think are important in the delivery of high-quality care. From there we help you to think about doing, and using, research, and finish by emphasizing the importance of evaluating nursing practice.

The first few chapters of the book focus on research used in everyday practice in order to:

- show you the link between research and advancing practice;
- draw your attention to key research studies that underpin essential aspects of practice: we have selected quality of life, dignity and pressure ulcer prevention and care to use as exemplars of where research undertaken by nurses has made a difference to the care that is delivered;
- show you what enthuses researchers and what it's like to be a researcher: we use short case studies from people working on some of these studies throughout this section to do this and to bring the text to life;
- emphasize how hard it is to implement changes to practice even when there is plenty of sound research evidence.

Later chapters focus more on the technicalities of doing and implementing research, addressing questions like:

- How do I ask a worthwhile question to research? (Chapter 5)
- What sort of research designs are there? (Chapter 6)
- How can I collect information to answer research questions? (Chapter 7)
- How can I analyse information to get an answer? (Chapter 7)
- If I want to do research, how do I get permission to do it? (Chapter 8)
- How do I go about telling other people about my research? (Chapter 9)

- How can I use research in my practice? (Chapter 10)
- How can I improve practice and evaluate care? (Chapter 11)

We anticipate that you will use this book in a number of ways. Some of you will just want to dip into it to try to answer specific questions or to find out more about research in the areas of practice that we have focused on. Others will read it right the way through in order to develop a more complete understanding of how to do research and how to develop research-based care. Throughout the book we have tried to encourage you to interact with the materials presented – we have exercises for you to do, topics for you to think about and summary boxes to help you understand quickly what each chapter has to offer you.

Once you have read this book we hope that you will be ready to take your knowledge of nursing research beyond the fundamentals presented here and read other, more detailed texts about research, quality improvement and practice development. But perhaps more importantly, we hope that you will want to implement the best research into your practice in order to provide your patients and their families and carers with the best possible care. Eventually, some of you may also end up as researchers, too – as we did!

Read on …

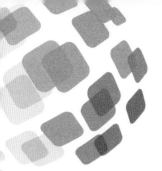

# Chapter 1

# Advancing practice through research

## ■ Introduction

This chapter discusses the drive for advancing practice using evidence and how research can help us to achieve this. We discuss why we need evidence-based care and what it means to provide it. We ask where evidence comes from and how we know which the best forms of evidence are before considering the need for research/research awareness, how to access research-based information and how to implement it into practice where appropriate.

We start from the premise that, as practitioners, we provide care for individual patients based on our knowledge and experience, modifying that care as our knowledge increases. While this undoubtedly enhances patient care it also raises questions about how we decide what care to provide or why we deliver different care to patients who experience similar symptoms or have the same illness. This is particularly important in healthcare today, with its relentless emphasis on 'evidence' and 'outcomes' (Department of Health (DH) 2010).

## ■ The evidence-based culture

Government expectations, the emphasis on clinical effectiveness and the increased scrutiny of healthcare mean that we must provide evidence-based care to help us justify not only *what* we do but also *how* and *why* we do it, and to account for our actions in terms of their efficacy, effectiveness and, increasingly, cost, demonstrating this using evidence-based clinical and patient-reported outcome measures (DH 2010).

> **Exercise 1.1  Demand drivers**
>
> Try to identify the drivers of the demand for evidence-based care and think about why this is central to healthcare practice. What are the benefits to patient care?

It would be easy to believe that this is 'new' – it is not! The idea of research-based practice was first introduced by the Briggs Committee on Nursing (Department of Health and Social Security 1972) and reinforced by McFarlane (1980), who emphasized the need to increase the science base of nursing because, historically, many aspects of care had little scientific basis but were based on tradition or anecdote; we rarely questioned practices, passed from nurse to nurse, and the quality of patient care varied considerably. This, combined with the inevitable variability in effectiveness, underlies the move towards evidence-based practice (EBP).

However, political, professional and societal pressures also drive the demand for EBP (McSherry *et al* 2006). Politically, it offers opportunities to save time and money, improve patient outcomes, reduce costs and standardize care; implicit in the NHS Plan (DH 2000), it is strongly linked to clinical governance and quality improvement (Elcoat 2000). McKenna *et al* (2004) believe it is 'one of the most important underlying principles in modern health care'.

It is a professional obligation because our Code of Conduct, Performance and Ethics (Nursing and Midwifery Council (NMC) 2008) states that nurses must 'deliver care based on the best available evidence' ensuring that 'any advice … is evidence based if you are suggesting healthcare products or services' as 'you are **personally** accountable for actions and omission in your practice and must **always** be able to **justify** your decisions' (author's emphasis) (see Table 1.1).

**Table 1.1** Excerpt: Code of Conduct, Performance and Ethics (NMC 2008)

| **Provide a high standard of practice and care at all times** |
| :--- |
| Use the best available evidence |
| • You must deliver care based on the best available evidence or best practice. |
| • You must ensure any advice you give is evidence based if you are suggesting healthcare products or services. |
| • You must ensure that the use of complementary or alternative therapies is safe and in the best interests of those in your care. |
| **Keep your skills and knowledge up to date** |
| • You must have the knowledge and skills for safe and effective practice when working without direct supervision. |
| • You must recognize and work within the limits of your competence. |
| • You must keep your knowledge and skills up to date throughout your working life. |

Societal factors also increase the need for EBP. Patients both receive care and consume a service and, lying at the heart of healthcare, must have access to the information they need to make choices about their care (DH 2010). This increased awareness of health and illness and the levels of care and support they should expect means that patients now expect the most appropriate and best treatment and the right to choose the care they receive (Berenholtz and Provonost 2003). Indeed, giving people more choice is an

NHS priority (DH 2010). Patients are increasingly well informed and willing to challenge professionals; nurses must be able to explain their actions.

This means that we must examine anecdotal and unsupported practices to develop our profession and protect patients from inappropriate and, occasionally, unsafe care. We must use evidence to substantiate our interventions and professional judgements (Rolfe 1998); EBP is not an 'optional extra' but central to everyday practice.

> **Exercise 1.2  Evidence-based practice**
>
> Write down your understanding of EBP and compare it with the material below.

## ■ What is evidence-based practice?

Evidence-based practice is a systematic approach that emphasizes the use of best evidence, clinical experience and patient preferences to make decisions about the care and treatment that will obtain the best patient outcomes by selecting interventions that have the greatest chance of success (Craig and Smyth 2007). It can be simply defined as 'the integration of best research evidence with clinical expertise, and patient values' (Sackett *et al* 2000). It has many benefits (see Table 1.2), promoting a systematic search for, and critical appraisal of, relevant evidence to answer clinical questions and guide

**Table 1.2**  Benefits of evidence-based practice (adapted from le May 1999)

| | |
|---|---|
| **For patients** | Improved care and reduced time wasted on inappropriate treatments |
| | Enhances consistency in care |
| | Increases understanding of investigations and treatment |
| | Increases confidence in practitioners and the NHS |
| **For clinical practitioners** | Actively involves them in determining the appropriateness and effectiveness of care |
| | Helps in redefining and/or changing practice where necessary |
| | Enhances quality of care |
| | Presents evidence of the benefits of practice to patients and carers |
| | Increases accountability for care provision |
| **For the NHS** | Enables consistent decision making |
| | Reduces variation in services |
| | Promotes cost-effectiveness |
| | Promotes integration of activities (e.g. research and development, clinical audit, continuing professional development) |
| | Increases accountability to the public for the service provided |

decisions about whether particular interventions are useful, based on evidence about what does and does not work (DH 1997). It is conscientious (deliberate, careful), explicit (clear that it is used) and judicious (well thought through), highlighting the importance of clinical expertise because 'without clinical expertise, practice risks becoming tyrannized by evidence but without best available evidence practice risks becoming rapidly out of date' (Sackett *et al* 1996).

This means that EBP, like nursing, promotes holistic care, taking account of patients' medical conditions and individual needs (Rolfe 1998) and acknowledging that evidence changes constantly as new knowledge becomes available. It offers a framework for care that relies on research and other evidence rather than only on nursing theory, experience or intuition (Scott and McSherry 2009). It may reduce the research–practice gap (Hutchinson and Johnston 2004) and improve the quality of professional decisions, showing that good clinical practice is based on using evidence that intervention A is helpful for treating condition B in patient C (Greenhalgh 1996). It involves a mixture of skills, such as critical thinking, to identify clinical questions and evaluate the findings, and 'technical' skills, like searching online resources and interpreting the material. Thus it combines our nursing knowledge with literature, research and technology to improve patient care and advance practice.

EBP comprises five steps (see Figure 1.1): asking questions, finding and evaluating evidence, determining the intervention and evaluation. It is not, therefore, unlike the nursing process with which you are familiar. The skill lies in asking the right question(s) (see Chapter 5), generating relevant evidence and using it appropriately to provide effective care.

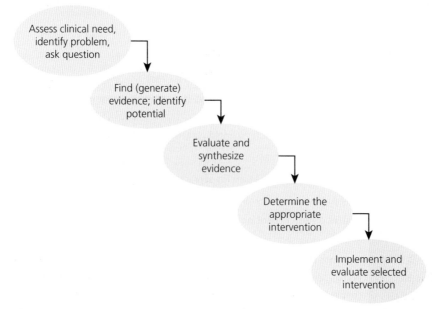

**Figure 1.1**  Implementing evidence-based practice

However, because EBP means acknowledging that clinical decisions are often associated with uncertainty, nurses can find it difficult even though 'perhaps the most important skill for any healthcare professional to master ... is the ability to recognise and handle clinical uncertainty ... presented by our patients in wards, outpatients, and in the consulting room, but also about one's own skill, expertise and knowledge base' (Kitson 1999). But it is only by acknowledging uncertainty, asking questions and balancing different sources of evidence to inform decision making that we can advance practice.

## Where does evidence come from?

Evidence is simply a piece of information that supports a conclusion; in healthcare, this typically refers to the effectiveness of interventions in achieving specific outcomes. However, although choosing the right evidence is important, this can be difficult as there are so many potential sources (see Table 1.3). We need to know what is meant by 'evidence', which form of evidence is 'best' and how we reach conclusions about its quality.

**Table 1.3**  Sources of evidence for nursing practice (adapted from le May 1999)

| Sources of evidence | Actions |
| --- | --- |
| **Research** | Search published and unpublished literature – original research (primary sources), reviews (secondary sources), clinical guidelines (e.g. NICE), published research-based standards of care |
| | Generate own evidence through research |
| **Experience (professional or general)** | Reflect on practice: articulate reflections, facilitate discussion, search the literature |
| **Theoretical experience (not research-based)** | Search the literature (published or unpublished), learn from others, facilitate discussions |
| **Evidence gathered from patients and/or their carers** | Search the literature for experiential writings and/or research findings, use audit data, levels of satisfaction and/or complaint, facilitate discussion and collaborative decision making |
| **Evidence passed on from role models and/or experts** | Facilitate discussion and observation, consult with experts. Search the literature for findings from consensus-reaching techniques (focus groups, Delphi surveys, nominal groups technique and consensus conferences) |
| **Evidence derived from policy documents** | Scrutinize documentation, facilitate discussion |

## Which evidence is 'best'?

There is little agreement in nursing about what 'good' evidence is (Jennings and Loan 2001), perhaps because the questions we ask relate not only to intervention(s) but also, for example, to how patients experience care, or nurse–patient relationships. 'Best evidence' refers to research based on a design most relevant to the question asked, likely to lead to reliable and valid findings and reduce the uncertainties that first led to the need for information (see Chapter 6).

These 'best' designs are sometimes considered using hierarchies of evidence (Thompson 2003), which offer a way of evaluating the reliability (or lack of potential bias) of research findings, giving insight into the perceived value of different research approaches (see Table 1.4). There are a number of such hierarchies focusing primarily on the effectiveness of interventions; they provide a simple way of estimating the trust we can place in research findings and/or recommendations.

**Table 1.4**  An example of a hierarchy of evidence

| Level | Description | Sources (examples) |
|---|---|---|
| One | Strong evidence from at least one systematic review or meta-analysis of well-designed randomized controlled trials (RCTs)<br><br>Multi-centre studies | The Cochrane Collaboration<br><br>Database of Abstracts of Reviews of Effects (DARE) |
| Two | Evidence from at least one RCT of appropriate size | Articles published in peer-reviewed journals |
| Three | Evidence from well-designed trials without randomization: cohort, time series or matched case-controlled studies | Articles published in peer-reviewed journals |
| Four | Evidence from well-designed non-experimental studies from more than one centre or research group | Articles published in peer-reviewed journals |
| Five | Opinions from respected authorities, based on clinical evidence, descriptive studies or reports from committees | NICE guidelines<br>Evidence-based local procedures and care pathways |
| Six | Professional opinions from colleagues or peers | Nursing colleagues or members of the multi-disciplinary team |

## Systematic reviews

When clinical decisions involve selecting a treatment/intervention from a range of choices, systematic reviews of good-quality randomized controlled trials are considered the most valid and reliable research evidence (Thompson 2003). These comprehensive literature reviews 'sum up' the evidence by synthesizing the results of relevant clinical research. Studies are screened for quality and the data synthesized so that the findings of many studies can be combined to make recommendations for care. Equally useful are meta-analyses, which pool the data from studies with related hypotheses; you can find these by doing a literature search.

Such reviews are valuable and present the current state of science, often resolving conflicting reports of the evidence. You can access them through databases such as the Cochrane Database of Systematic Reviews (www.thecochranelibrary.com). Systematic reviews of qualitative studies (meta-syntheses) are increasingly available.

### Randomized controlled trials

When we cannot find a review on a specific topic, we need to search for papers reporting independent randomized controlled trials (RCTs) using databases such as MEDLINE, the Cumulative Index of Nursing and Allied Health Literature (CINAHL) (**www.ebscohost.com/cinahl**), the National Guideline Clearinghouse (**www.guideline.gov**) or the Joanna Briggs Institute (**www.joannabriggs.edu.au**). RCTs are quantitative, comparative, controlled studies where people are randomly allocated to receive one of several clinical interventions, usually including the standard treatment (control).

However, though RCTs are highly regarded, they also have limitations. A single study, no matter how rigorous, relates to a single population under specific conditions so we cannot generalize it to the breadth and scope underlying nursing practice (Schutz *et al* 2008); neither will it explain *why* beneficial outcomes are achieved. RCTs tell us little about how patients feel about the intervention or its effects, or explore/explain factors important to nursing: how patients feel or experience treatment, whether it is acceptable to them or its impact on their quality of life (Britten 2010); individual needs, clinical aims and goals are unique. This means that the findings are rarely directly transferable to nursing; RCTs consider the science without the art (Adams 2010). EBP tries to balance the science and the art of nursing, combining them with patient preferences and clinical judgement. This balance is essential to define the best practice for nursing. You will find an example of this in Box 6.2, page 65.

## Other sources of evidence

Less well-regarded as sources of evidence are trials that don't include randomization and which may not be controlled (e.g. cohort, time series or case-controlled studies), while the least reliable and valid forms are professional opinions, descriptive studies or committee reports. Though expert opinion is the lowest level of acceptable evidence, nurses place higher value on it for decision making than any other source of information (Thompson *et al* 2001), but if it is the best evidence available, it may still meet the criteria for EBP.

## Criteria for best evidence

Though hierarchies of evidence have been developed to enable different research approaches to be ranked according to the validity of their findings (Evans 2003), considering the effectiveness, appropriateness and feasibility of interventions, they also have limitations as they focus on evaluating the effectiveness of interventions and overlook qualitative studies, policies/guidance and clinical experience; they do not indicate how to manage individual patients or address specific clinical questions. Thus, existing hierarchies may not help us to determine the applicability of evidence to specific clinical circumstances. In any case, qualitative approaches may provide the best answer to some clinical questions, and so offer the best evidence.

The criteria for best evidence, therefore, include not only its scientific rigour but also its relevance and applicability to individual patients and clinical settings. Once evidence is identified, it must be evaluated, focusing particularly on its validity, findings and application (see Chapter 10). This means that evidence for nursing stretches beyond particular types of research (Jennings and Loan 2001); all research designs have their purpose and associated strengths, weaknesses and limitations (see Chapter 6). The important thing is that the right research design has been used to answer the question asked. It is only when clinically relevant research, clinical expertise and patient choice are considered together that the best evidence is produced, leading to effective, individualized patient care (Mulhall 1998; Kitson 1999).

## ■ The need for research and research awareness

EBP in nursing has been defined as 'a problem-solving approach to clinical practice that integrates a systematic search for, and critical appraisal of, the most relevant evidence to answer a burning clinical question, one's own clinical expertise, patient preferences and values' (Melnyk and Fineout-Overholt 2005); it might also include generating our own evidence through research and, indeed, nurses are increasingly doing this – it is not new! Nursing has been a research-focused profession for more than 40 years and nurses' education fosters a belief in practices that are research-based (Leufer and Cleary-Holdforth 2009). Nurses constantly seek answers to important questions that can lead to healthier, more effective and safer experiences for patients and their families; they have made, and will continue to make, a huge contribution to patient outcomes by engaging in research and, through this, advancing practice.

This is implicit in our Code of Professional Conduct; we not only have a professional obligation to EBP but also to develop our knowledge (NMC 2008) (see Table 1.1, page 6); research helps us to fulfil both these objectives. This does not mean that we should all conduct research, but we must be research aware, able to access information about service developments, innovations and research findings, and able to interpret and critically appraise this information so as to implement and evaluate practice based on the best available evidence (McSherry et al 2006). This helps us to subject the 'art' of nursing to scientific scrutiny and substantiate claims of effective practice (Thompson 1998). Unless we integrate research with practice we will be unable to build a meaningful knowledge base to enable the delivery of truly evidence-based care (Clarke and Procter 1999).

## What is nursing research?

Nursing research is practice- or discipline-orientated, focusing primarily on clinical care or patients' responses to actual or potential health problems. Its purposes are to:

- promote the development of nursing knowledge;
- generate information which helps to define the unique role of nursing;
- help us to demonstrate professional accountability;
- enable us to make more informed decisions, facilitate evaluation of practice and articulate our role in care delivery;
- support evidence-based practice;
- improve/advance patient care.

Nursing research is a general term used to describe studies designed to find answers to nursing questions, solve a problem or validate nursing knowledge using an objective and systematic search for understanding. It is directed towards establishing the effectiveness of interventions, gaining knowledge that directly or indirectly influences nursing practice, or analysing phenomena (things) of importance to nursing or patients. It complements practice by combining art and science; identifying appropriate questions, which can be answered by research, relies on both creativity and curiosity (Thompson 1998).

Research begins with a clearly defined goal or aim, usually in the form of a hypothesis or question, which helps us to decide the best way to address the problem (see Chapters 5 and 6). Examples include trials to investigate the safety or effectiveness of new interventions or compare two treatments or methods of care, studies designed to investigate how a procedure or intervention could be improved, to explain how patients cope with illness or understand particular procedures or conditions.

This range of possible studies arises because nursing involves many different aspects, illustrated by this definition of nursing: 'diagnosis and treatment of human responses to actual or potential health problems' (American Nurses' Association 1980). Since such responses may be physical, biological, emotional or social we may need to study complex situations or consider multiple factors and use a variety of approaches; there is no single way to 'do' nursing research. The important things are that the science of nursing evolves from, and responds to, the needs of practice, and research priorities emerge from nurses who are caring for patients (Cullum 1998).

That said, nursing must take a broad approach to generating and finding evidence, sometimes 'borrowing' evidence from other disciplines (Clarke 1997) while maintaining a nursing focus. Though other disciplines may provide useful evidence, they rarely look at the problem or findings in the same way, thus offering only limited solutions to nursing questions. Patients are more than a collection of signs and symptoms or diseases; nurses provide care that takes individuals and their needs into account. This holistic perspective necessitates a broader approach considering potential relationships between individuals and their disease or illness. What is important is that the research designs adopted reflect the diversity of practice and incorporate scientific, social and behavioural science as appropriate. The outcomes of nursing research may, therefore, lie in a number of areas: clinical, functional, satisfaction and/or cost.

*Clinical outcomes* include disease-specific indicators, such as wound healing, pain, or nutritional markers (e.g. weight gain/loss), level of complications or other factors related specifically to the patient's condition. These can be systematically measured to provide useful information about interventions or approaches to care.

*Functional outcomes* include such issues as the patient's physical and psychological condition in terms of, for example, ability to take part in activities of daily living, exercise capacity, well-being or quality of life. Many nursing interventions can affect such factors; selecting between them can be achieved using indicators like these.

*Patient satisfaction* is an important outcome, particularly as they are consumers of services as well as recipients of care. Satisfaction can be measured, using surveys or interviews, providing valuable information about nursing interventions and care. As key stakeholders in healthcare, patients' views are crucial to gaining understanding of anything from the quality of service provision to the effectiveness of treatment (McKenna 2011). Patient-reported outcomes offer a way of gathering their views.

*Cost* of care is an increasingly important consideration.Measurement includes issues such as length of stay, readmission rates and costs of equipment and/or resources. This enables us to distinguish between interventions which are equally effective in, for example, preventing infection or promoting wound healing, enabling the cost–benefit to be analysed; this should include consideration of the human costs.

Taken together, these outcomes provide us with information about different approaches to care or alternative interventions and, with patient preferences/choices, enable us to select the most appropriate care for individuals. Using the same approaches to measurement across many studies allows us to compare the findings across different settings and patient samples, thus strengthening the evidence.

## Difficulties and barriers to nursing research

Nurses often see research as irrelevant to their daily work, perhaps because searching for and evaluating evidence reduces the time available for patient care. But EBP is now embedded in healthcare and is not going to go away. In fact, research and EBP offer us opportunities to demonstrate our contribution to clinical effectiveness. 'Research is not a luxury for the academic, but a tool for developing the quality of nursing decisions, prescriptions and actions. Whether as clinicians, educators, managers or researchers, we have a research responsibility; neglect of that responsibility should be classified as professional negligence' (McFarlane 1984).

That said, there are barriers to research in practice (see Chapter 10), including time constraints and lack of managerial support and encouragement (Gerrish and Clayton 2004), together with low staffing levels and negative attitudes to research (Hundley *et al* 2000). The way research is presented can also limit its accessibility to practitioners; it can be difficult to interpret the academic style used in many research papers, not surprising when we remember that most researchers write for other researchers, not for practitioners. Thus much research is never seen by the nurses who could use it and researchers are frustrated that their valuable work is not widely circulated (Shuttleworth 2011). Researchers could help by publishing in the journals that clinicians read and emphasizing their relevance for practice.

### Accessing research-based information

We can obtain information in many ways, including through computer searching or journals focusing on evidence to guide practice (e.g. *Evidence-Based Nursing*), supported by national initiatives, such as the Cochrane Collaboration, NHS Evidence and Clinical Knowledge Summaries and the NHS Centre for Reviews and Dissemination, which produce and maintain systematic reviews and/or a core database of up-to-date evidence of the effects of healthcare.

Research clearly has the potential to inform us not only about nursing but also about relevant physical and scientific issues, increasing 'available knowledge by the discovery of new factors or relationships' (Macleod Clark and Hockey 1989), 'generate(ing) and refine(ing) clinical nursing interventions' (Rolfe 1994) and so advancing practice. It therefore enables us to subject the art of nursing to scientific scrutiny and substantiate claims to provide effective and efficient practice (Thompson 1998). This is essential if we are to develop a body of knowledge and generate theories to underpin and advance practice – we must identify areas of concern and design our own research to investigate them. Without this, nursing will not evolve and practice will remain unchanged.

## ▪ Overview: implementing evidence and research into practice (Figure 1.2)

The government is committed to the promotion and conduct of research as a core NHS activity, seeing it as vital in providing the new knowledge needed to improve health outcomes, reduce inequalities and identify new ways of preventing, diagnosing and treating disease (DH 2010). Despite this, it is increasingly recognized that the full potential of research to improve healthcare practice has not yet been realized and its benefits have been slow to become part of routine practice (Wilson *et al* 2010).

Lack of research awareness has, traditionally, been a barrier to utilization, yet this is the first step in translating it into practice. Important also is individual motivation towards implementing change together with practitioners' belief in themselves and their ability to implement it. Balancing the benefits of change against the costs, both financial and personal, is one step towards the likelihood of change (see Chapter 10). Research and evidence are essential in attempts to achieve this.

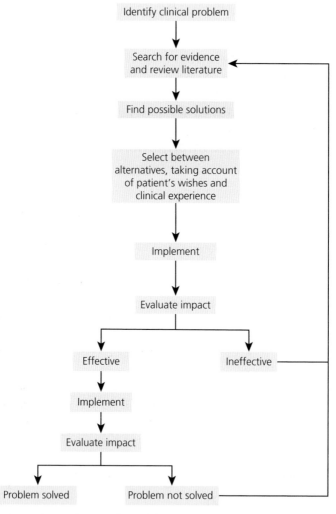

**Figure 1.2** Implementing evidence and research into practice

**Exercise 1.4  Research in practice**

Think about how you might be able to use research in your practice and what the benefits of doing so could be.

Using research and evidence in practice (see Chapter 10) requires us to:

- find relevant research/evidence by searching the literature and/or asking experts;
- assess the quality of that research/evidence;
- determine which evidence provides the best approach to care, is appropriate to the situation and the patient, and can be provided by the organization;
- make necessary changes to practice to incorporate the evidence;
- evaluate the impact of that evidence on the care being provided;
- keep up to date and change practice accordingly.

As a cornerstone of healthcare, nurses are driven by compassion and personal commitment to ensure that patients and their families receive the highest quality of care. Asking the 'what', 'how' and 'why' questions, and answering these by engaging in research and implementing EBP, are ways through which we can contribute to innovation and excellence in patient care and advance practice.

## References

Adams JS. Utilizing evidence-based research and practice to support the infusion alliance. *Journal of Infusion Nursing.* 2010; **33**(5): 273–277.

American Nurses' Association. *Nursing: A Social Policy Statement.* 1980; Kansas City, MO: ANA.

Berenholtz S, Provonost PJ. Barriers to translating evidence into practice. *Current Opinion in Critical Care.* 2003; **9**(4): 321–325.

Britten N. Qualitative research and the take-up of evidence-based practice. *Journal of Research in Nursing.* 2010; **15**(6): 537–544.

Clarke C, Procter S. Practice development: ambiguity in research and practice. *Journal of Advanced Nursing.* 1999; **30**(4): 975–982.

Clarke J. Evidence-based practice: a retrograde step? The importance of pluralism in evidence generation for the practice of health care. *Journal of Clinical Nursing.* 1997; **6**(1): 175–178.

Craig JV, Smyth RL (eds). *The Evidence-Based Practice Manual for Nurses.* Second edition. 2007; Edinburgh: Churchill Livingstone Elsevier.

Cullum N. Evidence-based practice. *Nursing Management.* 1998; **5**(3): 32–35.

Department of Health. *The New NHS: Modern, Dependable.* 1997; London: The Stationery Office.

Department of Health. *The NHS Plan: A plan for investment, a plan for reform.* 2000; London: The Stationery Office.

Department of Health. *Equity and Excellence: Liberating the NHS* (Cm7881). 2010; London: The Stationery Office. Available from **www.dh.gov.uk/en/Publicationsandstatistics/ Publications/PublicationsPolicyAndGuidance/DH_117353.**

Department of Health and Social Security. *Report of the Committee on Nursing* (Cmd5115, Briggs Report). 1972; London: DHSS.

Elcoat D. Clinical governance in action; key issues in clinical effectiveness. *Professional Nurse*. 2000; **18**(10): 822–823.

Evans D. Hierarchy of evidence: a framework for ranking evidence evaluating healthcare interventions. *Journal of Clinical Nursing*. 2003; **12**(1): 77–84.

Gerrish K, Clayton J. Promoting evidence-based practice: an organizational approach. *Journal of Nursing Management*. 2004; **12**(2): 114–123.

Greenhalgh T. 'Is my practice evidence-based?' should be answered in qualitative, as well as quantitative terms. *British Medical Journal*. 1996; **313**(**7063**): 957–958.

Hundley V, Milne J, Leighton-Beck L, Graham W, Fitzmaurice A. Raising research awareness among midwives and nurses: does it work? *Journal of Advanced Nursing*. 2000; **31**(1): 78–88.

Hutchinson AM, Johnston L. Bridging the divide: a survey of nurses' opinions regarding barriers to, and facilitators of, research utilization in the practice setting. *Journal of Clinical Nursing*. 2004; **13**(3): 304–315.

Jennings BM, Loan LA. Misconceptions among nurses about evidence-based practice. *Image: Journal of Nursing Scholarship*. 2001; **33**(2): 121–127.

Kitson A. Research utilization: current issues, questions, and debates. *Canadian Journal of Nursing Research*. 1999; **31**(1): 13–22.

le May A. *Evidence-based Practice. Nursing Times Clinical Monographs No 2*. 1999; London: Nursing Times Books Ltd.

Leufer T, Cleary-Holdforth J. Evidence-based practice: improving patient outcomes. *Nursing Standard*. 2009; **23**(32): 35–39.

McFarlane J. *Accountability*. Report of the Royal College of Nursing. 1980; London: RCN.

McFarlane J. Foreword. In: DFS Cormack (ed.). *The Research Process in Nursing*. 1984; Oxford: Blackwell.

McKenna HP, Ashton S, Keeney S. Barriers to evidence-based practice in primary care. *Journal of Advanced Nursing*. 2004; **45**(2): 178–189.

McKenna SP. Measuring patient-reported outcomes: moving beyond misplaced common sense to hard science. *BMC Medicine*. 2011; **9**(86): doi:10.1186/1741-7015-9-86.

Macleod Clark J, Hockey L. *Further Research for Nursing*. 1989; London: Scutari.

McSherry R, Artley A, Holloran J. Research awareness: an important factor for evidence-based practice? *Worldviews on Evidence-Based Nursing*. 2006; **3**(3): 103–115.

Melnyk B, Fineout-Overholt E. *Evidence-Based Practice in Nursing and Healthcare: A guide to best practice*. 2005; Philadelphia, PA: Lippincott, Williams and Wilkins.

Mulhall A. Nursing, research and the evidence. *Evidence Based Nursing*. 1998; **1**(1): 4–6.

Nursing and Midwifery Council. *The Code: Standards of conduct, performance and ethics for nurses and midwives*. 2008; London: NMC.

Rolfe G. Towards a new model of nursing research. *Journal of Advanced Nursing*. 1994; **19**(5): 969–975.

Rolfe G. The theory–practice gap in nursing: from research-based practice to practitioner-based research. *Journal of Advanced Nursing*. 1998; **28**(3): 672–679.

Sackett DL, Rosenberg WM, Gray JA, Haynes RB, Richardson WS. Evidence-based medicine: what it is and what it is not. *British Medical Journal*. 1996; **312**(7023): 71–72.

Sackett DL, Straus SE, Richardson WS, Rosenberg W, Haynes RB. *Evidence-based Medicine: How to practice and teach EBM*. Second edition. 2000; Edinburgh: Churchill Livingstone.

Schutz LE, Rivers KO, Ratusnik DL. The role of external validity in evidence-based practice for rehabilitation. *Rehabilitation Psychology*. 2008; **53**(3): 294–302.

Scott K, McSherry R. Evidence-based nursing: clarifying the concepts for nurses in practice. *Journal of Clinical Nursing*. 2009; **18**(8): 1085–1095.

Shuttleworth A. A lot of research is barely seen by the nurses who could use it. *Nursing Times*. 2011; available from **www.nursingtimes.net/5033548.article?referrer=el8**.

Thompson C. Clinical experience as evidence in evidence-based practice. *Journal of Advanced Nursing*. 2003; **43**(3): 230–237.

Thompson C, McCaughan D, Cullum N, Sheldon TA, Mulhall A, Thompson DR. Research information in nurses' clinical decision-making: what is useful? *Journal of Advanced Nursing*. 2001; **36**(3): 376–388.

Thompson DR. The art and science of research in clinical nursing. In: B Roe and C Webb (eds). *Research and Development in Clinical Nursing Practice*. 1998; London: Whurr Publishers Ltd.

Wilson P, Pettigrew M, Calnan MW, Nazareth I. Disseminating research findings: what should researchers do? A systematic scoping review of conceptual frameworks. *Implementation Science*. 2010; **5**(91): doi:10.1186/1748-5908-5-91.

# Chapter 2

# Quality of life research: implications for nursing

---

**Box 2.1    My research into quality of life**

My research into quality of life (QL) was stimulated by working in oncology wards and, strange as it may seem, my concern over patients' nutritional status. At that time we were aware that malnutrition caused many deleterious effects on patients' physical and psychological condition – and many patients with cancer developed malnutrition. These effects led me to think that there could be a relationship between nutrition and quality of life and I wanted to investigate this in affected patients. This became the topic of my PhD at the University of Surrey, meaning that I needed to search the literature to try to establish what this 'thing' called quality of life was. Using this information, I finally defined QL as 'an abstract and complex term representing individual responses to the physical, mental and social factors contributing to "normal" daily living'. As you will see later, there are reasons why this seems somewhat vague.

Using this definition I (then) believed that it was possible to design some form of questionnaire to measure QL and take individual circumstances into account. This I did and you can find an account of this in Holmes and Dickerson (1987). My work continued and I completed my PhD (Quality of Life, Nutrition and Cancer 1989), finding that there was indeed a relationship between QL and malnutrition in that, as patients' nutritional status declined, so too did their QL. This, sadly, remains the case even today as scientists are not yet able to reverse the nutritional impact of many types of cancer.

I have maintained my interest in QL since the 1980s and have conducted many studies, most recently a project focused on QL in an internet chat room (Holmes 2006). However, while the topic remains fascinating, a definition of QL remains elusive, as you will see. But I continue to try and am currently involved in a study trying to define QL in the UK population at large.

# ■ Introduction

Rapid social change and developments in medicine and technology have increased concern about patient well-being, acknowledging the psychosocial consequences of disease and illness, leading to wider consideration of the 'human costs' of illness (Macduff 2000) and recognition that patients' perspectives of outcomes are as valid as those of clinicians (Leplege and Hunt 1997). Assessing quality of life is, therefore, increasingly advocated as a way of incorporating patients' and users' perspectives of their experience. At the same time, nurses often talk about maintaining patients' QL as many of the anticipated outcomes of care relate to improvements in QL (Harrison *et al* 1996). Parse (1994) explicitly stated that this is the goal of nursing; by understanding the factors influencing patients' QL, we can intervene and have a positive impact (Mandzuk and McMillan 2005).

For these reasons, QL is now an important patient-reported outcome used in formulating healthcare objectives, guidelines and policies, evaluating not only the effects of illness and the impact of nursing but also services, and comparing equivalent therapies with similar effects on morbidity/mortality but different effects on QL (Rotstein *et al* 2000). It is an end-point for randomized controlled trials and used to justify resource allocation and contract specification (Ager 2002; Moons *et al* 2006); research findings are often described in terms of QL. 'Expected QL' may be used in deciding whether treatment for life-threatening conditions is given or withdrawn (Pellegrino 2000).

# ■ QL is a 'hot topic'

For many economic, social and political reasons, notions of QL, well-being and the 'good life' are now important in every realm of service delivery and public policy making. QL has a high public profile and is a widely used outcome in not only healthcare but also education, social services and, increasingly, the public sector, particularly with regard to supporting local communities. Even politicians try to convince us that their policies will improve the nation's QL; indeed, the current UK government emphasizes 'happiness', and at the end of 2010, the Office for National Statistics (ONS) launched a debate on national well-being to develop measures of people's subjective well-being, experiences, feelings and perceptions of how their lives are going (see Box 2.2).

This seems to have arisen due to the New Economics Foundation's (NEF) report, 'National accounts of well-being' (2009), which called for regular, systematic collection of such information to be published as it is the subjective dimensions which have, to date, been lacking in national assessments.

I believe this emphasis on QL is a cause for concern due to the many different perspectives on QL and lack of consensus on its definition and meaning. Even the NEF

| Box 2.2 | Measuring national well-being |
|---|---|

To develop measures of national well-being, intended to cover the QL of people in the UK, the environment and sustainability and the country's economic performance, the ONS needed to find out what people think 'national well-being' means and how they would use the new measures. A consultation, launched in November 2010 and closed in April 2011, asked people, organizations, businesses and government across the UK: what makes our lives worthwhile? What things improve, or detract from, well-being? To help people decide, the ONS provided a list of things that they 'know' affect national well-being, such as:

- income and wealth;
- job satisfaction and economic security;
- ability to have a say on local and national issues;
- having good connections with friends and relatives;
- present and future conditions of the environment;
- crime;
- health;
- education and training;
- personal and cultural activities, including caring and volunteering.

**www.ons.gov.uk/ons/about-ons/consultations/closed-consultations/measuring-national-well-being/index.html**

and the government use different terms interchangeably – quality of life, well-being and happiness – though there is no certainty that they are the 'same thing'. Indeed, my research suggests that people believe happiness contributes to QL; if they aren't happy, their QL is poor (Holmes 2006). Though QL is something 'everyone' understands, it is also something few can define.

## Meaning and use of quality of life

The literature about QL – or health-related QL (HRQL) – has increased substantially in the past 30–40 years. But in 1983, when I first became interested in QL, this was rare. Bardelli and Saracci (1978), for example, reported that QL was measured in less than 4% of clinical trials, but Jones *et al* (1987) found more than 200 papers reporting QL data between 1978 and 1980. Now there are thousands every year; it's almost impossible to find clinical papers that don't make at least passing reference to QL.

The term 'quality of life' is, therefore, widely used and it seems to be assumed that 'everyone' knows what it means. Yet the reality may be very different. Try this.

### Exercise 2.1   Quality of life

Work out what quality of life means to you and what things (factors) are important in determining your QL. Now ask friends, colleagues or members of your family. Try to include people of different ages, genders and, if possible, from different cultural backgrounds. Then ask them to put the factors determining QL in rank order (most important first).

Compare their responses with yours, noting any similarities and differences. We'll return to the ranking later in the chapter.

Exercise 2.1 is likely to have shown you that people define QL very differently; while there may be similarities, different things are important to different people. Despite this, use of QL in healthcare has grown exponentially over time (Moons *et al* 2006). Not surprisingly, there are multiple definitions reflecting these differing perspectives – you can see some examples in Box 2.3.

### Box 2.3    Some definitions of quality of life over time

'The possession of resources necessary to the satisfaction of individual needs, wants and desires, participation in activities enabling personal development and self-actualisation and satisfactory comparison between oneself and others.' (Shin and Johnson 1978)

'Satisfaction, contentment, happiness, fulfilment and the ability to cope … difference, at a particular period of time, between the hopes and expectations of the individual and present experience.' (Calman 1984)

'The functional effect of an illness and its consequent therapy … as perceived by the patient.' (Schipper *et al*, 1990)

'Sense of well-being that stems from satisfaction or dissatisfaction with the areas of life that are important to him or her.' (Ferrans 1990)

'An individual's perception of their position in life in the context of the culture and value systems in which they live and in relation to their goals, expectations, standards and concerns … affected in a complex way by … health, psychological state, level of independence, social relationships and their relationship to salient features of their environment.' (World Health Organisation 1995)

'How an individual perceives his own life, in light of the cultural context and values of his environment, aims, expectations and worries.' (Bonomi *et al* 2000)

'How the individual's well-being may be impacted by a certain disease, or disability, or a disorder.' (National Center for Chronic Disease Prevention and Health Promotion 2011)

What Box 2.3 shows is that, like the definitions given by your friends and family, interpretations of QL vary and lack precision and specificity. Even in healthcare, QL is poorly defined, having many interpretations, and few researchers have asked patients directly about the factors they think constitute QL. When patients *are* involved, they are usually asked about the impact of illness on their lives or behaviour but not about things that are *important in* their lives.

Researchers have attempted to differentiate HRQL from that arising from other areas of life covering five broad concepts: duration of life, functional status, impairment, health perceptions and opportunities (Patrick and Bergner 1990). This limits notions of QL to aspects of disease and/or treatment and subjective experience relating directly/ indirectly to health or impairment associated with specific diseases or the effect of treatment (Carr *et al* 2001). However, while health professionals believe that health includes physical, psychological and social well-being, they rarely consider spiritual and environmental aspects of human experience, yet nursing involves caring for the whole person, not only selected parts.

While Farquhar (1995) suggested that such difficulties arise because QL is a multi-disciplinary term, Keith (2001) argues that this is because QL cannot be precisely defined. What do you think?

Nevertheless, it seems probable that we can make some assumptions about QL in that it is likely to represent responses to the physical, mental, environmental and social factors contributing to 'normal' daily living. But the literature shows us that there are significant differences in perceptions between different groups of people which perhaps reflect the different populations involved, suggesting that potential components of QL are as varied as those who identify them and indicating its individual nature.

Other important factors that may also influence perceptions of QL are gender and age (Spiroch *et al* 2000) and culture. It is known that different cultural groups emphasize different aspects of QL (Scott *et al* 2008), suggesting that the generality of the concept we assume when undertaking assessment may affect the findings due to the way those from different cultures interpret QL and health. Indeed, Leininger (1994) provided examples from five different cultural groups to illustrate how QL is culturally constituted.

### Exercise 2.2  Interpretations of QL

Review Leininger's paper (Quality of life from a transcultural nursing perspective, *Nursing Science Quarterly*, 1994; 7: 22–28) and identify how different cultures interpret QL. Think about how this might influence your practice.

This shows that we need to consider the individual nature of QL rather than judging it by 'our' standards. We may all share the basic components of QL, but we may vary in the emphasis we place on them (Dalkey *et al* 1972). This means that, beyond core items, other items are likely to be more or less relevant to specific people (Sprangers 2002). In the same way that determinants of QL vary, so may the importance we attach to them according to individual expectations and aspirations (Carr and Higginson 2001); as QL is dynamic (Haas 1999) and ever-changing (Moons *et al* 2006), they may also change with time as we gain new experiences and knowledge. Thus 'knowing an individual's QOL at one time may not accurately predict his or her QOL at a subsequent time' (King *et al* 1997).

---

### Exercise 2.3  Comparisons

Now return to the information you collected earlier and look at the rankings your friends and family applied to the factors determining QL. Again, compare these with yours and note any similarities and differences. What does this suggest to you?

---

The information you've gained from the exercises may highlight another difficulty associated with QL: that of deciding which components are most important and how/if these should be weighted. Some people think that individuals can't compare the different domains, or that they can't be compared, while others incorporate weightings derived from the general population or from other samples of patients. However, since interpretations vary, even within the same people at different times (Hickey *et al* 1996), this probably doesn't reflect individual values which, like priorities, may change according to circumstances and experience (e.g. ageing, chronic illness). There may also be differences between different groups of patients, known as within- or between-patient variation (Carr and Higginson 2001).

Yet, despite these difficulties, many studies have tried to quantify and/or compare QL across patient groups. Such studies are often confounded by what is called the 'disability paradox'. Patients with significant health/functional problems or intrusive and clearly distressing symptoms do not necessarily have the QL scores you would expect them to have (e.g. Allbrecht and Devlieger 1999; Skevington 1999), perhaps reflecting changes in the criteria used to evaluate their lives following illness or disability (Sprangers and Schwartz 1999).

The fact that QL is so complex means that many authors duck the question and don't define QL at all but refer instead to its 'abstract' or 'subjective' nature; in other words, QL 'is what the researchers want it to be' (Bergner 1989 p150). Though you can understand this, it means that researchers are likely to study specific facets and dimensions; rather than provide explicit definition they will operationalize (use) QL in ways relevant to their work, making it difficult to compare the results of different studies. If you look back at the definition given in Box 2.1 (page 21) you can see that I, too, ducked the question, referring to QL as an 'abstract and complex term'.

Authors may, alternatively, use factors that are related to QL as proxies for it (e.g. performance status (www.qoltech.co.uk), subjective well-being (Andrews and Whitney 1976), 'sickness impact' (Bergner *et al* 1981), anxiety and depression (Zigmund and Snaith 1983) or 'symptom distress' (e.g. McCorkle and Young 1978)), though it isn't clear that they represent QL. Symptom reports, for example, don't relate to objective measures of physiological abnormality (Wilson and Cleary 1995), so we must question their reliability as indicators of QL. Not surprisingly, Evers (2003) suggested that we must distinguish QL from other 'things' that may be used as indicators of it. Objective measures may, however, provide indicators of physical condition, providing important knowledge for nursing.

This failure to clearly define what is being measured or talked about is important because, as we have seen, QL is widely used yet 'differences in meaning can lead to profound differences in outcomes for research, clinical practice, and allocation of healthcare resources' (Ferrans 1996 p294). Current studies using QL as an outcome measure are difficult to interpret and it's difficult to compare findings between studies, leading to doubt as to whether QL can be defined as a meaningful or enduring phenomenon (Hannestad 1990). Definition may be as simple as 'what you think of your life' or, like pain, QL is 'what the patient says it is' at the time when they say so (Holmes 2006).

## ■ Implications for nursing

This may cause you to ask whether it is worth using QL as an outcome measure. The answer is a resounding 'Yes!' because 'quality of life always matters to the patient' (Cohen *et al* 1996) and, if it matters to the patient, then it matters to us. Instead of losing our concern for patients' QL we should redouble our efforts to understand it; it is only by continued research and dialogue that we can move towards a definition of QL for nursing (King *et al* 1997).

In fact, nurses have made important contributions to understanding QL which has been examined in people experiencing particular illnesses, such as cancer (e.g. Holmes and Dickerson 1987). However, the many disciplinary perspectives of QL, and the lack of consensus about its meaning, have had limited success. This is complicated by the fact that nurses often try to analyse the concept from a social science rather than a nursing perspective, which, though useful, doesn't really help to develop nursing knowledge (Plummer and Molzahn 2009). That has still to come – a challenge for nurses as they develop their skills in research.

In the meantime, let's think about how we can use the idea of QL in practice. We already know that this is a central goal for nursing (Parse 1994), guiding the art of practice, so we must find ways of making the research useful to us.

---

**Exercise 2.4  Assessing QL**

How do you think nurses could use assessment of QL in their day-to-day practice? Can you see any ways in which improving understanding of QL could enhance the care you provide?

The literature tells us that the many aspects of QL are intertwined and can't be divided into discrete parts – reflecting holism and helping us to understand the inherent indivisibility of life and its quality (Phillips 1995). However it is defined, QL indicates individual life experience and determines how we feel. The environment (context) in which we have that experience is also important, having implications for care provision.

Potential benefits of using QL in practice are that patients' problems are identified and addressed and that treatment decisions are based on their priorities and preferences. Neugarten *et al* (1961) stated that 'individuals can be the only proper judge of their wellbeing' and von Essen and Sjoden (1993) that 'only the patient can know what the outsider must infer or speculate about', emphasizing the importance of asking patients how they feel if we are to understand their subjective experience (Spiroch *et al* 2000). In other words, we need to find out what's important to them. Using QL measures thus helps to ensure that treatment and evaluation focus on patients rather than on disease. They can be used to screen for and prioritize potential problems, facilitate communication, identify preferences and monitor changes or response to treatment (Higginson and Carr 2001).

For example, my research into QL in cancer (Holmes and Dickerson 1987) showed that scrutinizing completed questionnaires made it possible to identify areas of particular concern to individual patients, offering a useful way through which counselling could be initiated once problems had been identified. I had not set out to do this, but the study highlighted a number of areas where care could be improved. These included elements of communication and symptom distress which, at times, seemed to be closely related. For example, patients reported feeling isolated due to an inability to discuss their anxieties with nurses because they were 'too busy to waste time talking to me'. Symptom distress related to two aspects: pain and changes in appearance.

Pain can be isolating – sufferers feel 'separated' by their feelings and discomfort. The negative correlation between pain and the failure to communicate with nurses may indicate failure to identify the need for effective measures to relieve pain, enhance patient comfort and, therefore, QL. However, the problem causing most concern was changes in appearance, which were closely related to nausea, tiredness, concentration and mood. This is useful knowledge (evidence) for practice, providing guidance for appropriate interventions.

The first steps are, therefore, to understand the potential impact of patients' illness on QL and identify likely problems. This has been studied in various medical conditions such as breast cancer (e.g. Fallowfield 1995), chronic lung disease (e.g. Leidy and Coughlen 1998), congestive heart failure (e.g. Guyatt 1993), asthma (e.g. Rothman and Revicki 1993) and palliative care (e.g. Higginson and McCarthy 1994), helping to identify where supportive or symptomatic care is needed.

It is also important to know how much involvement patients want in decision making about their care; treatment decisions can't be based on patients' choices if we don't know what they are. A study in breast cancer, for example, showed that fewer than 50 per cent of women achieved their desired level of involvement, thus reducing their QL (Degner *et al* 1997). Since it is expected that patients have access to the information needed to make choices about their care (DH 2010), awareness of the levels of care and support they should receive have increased; patients now expect the most appropriate and best treatment and the right to choose their care (Berenholtz and Provonost 2003). Engaging in mutual goal setting between nurses and patients significantly improves QL (Scott *et al* 2004). That said, patients can't always imagine all the aspects of care about which they should have been informed (Jacobs 2000) so we may have to guide them.

Patient expectations are equally important, as Koller *et al* (2005) illustrated, showing that those expecting a cure from cancer treatment had significantly better QL before therapy while those anticipating pain relief achieved significantly lower scores; when patients in either group realized their expectations weren't fulfilled, QL was particularly low. Thus honesty and effective management of expectations are important. This again is useful evidence for practice but can be challenging for nurses who, it appears, want to be diplomatic, believing that patients and their families can't handle the truth using 'white lies' to 'protect' them and avoid dishonesty (Malloch 2001). These examples illustrate the importance of issues related to patients' QL and of treating patients as individuals.

So, does it matter if we can't define QL? Yes, of course it does if we're talking about populations or patient groups, but if we're talking about individuals, this may be less important. If we're providing holistic and patient-centred care – as we should – our care and interventions can be tailored to the needs of the individual.

We are morally obliged to respect the individuality and uniqueness of our patients (e.g. Thompson *et al* 2000) and this is known to enhance their QL (Stewart *et al* 2000; Annells *et al* 2001). This shows the value of research into QL and nursing and how, by adopting a holistic approach, we can enhance our practice, making our care truly patient-centred.

## ■ Further reading

Draper P. *Nursing Perspectives on Quality of Life.* 1997; London: Routledge.
Rapley M. *Quality of Life Research: A critical introduction.* 2003; London: Sage Publications Ltd.

## ■ References

Ager A. Quality of life assessment in critical context. *Journal of Applied Research in Intellectual Disabilities.* 2002; **15**(4): 369–376.
Allbrecht GL, Devlieger PJ. The disability paradox: high quality of life against all odds. *Social Science and Medicine.* 1999; **48**(8): 977–988.

Andrews FM, Whitney SB. *Social Indicators of Well-being: America's perception of life quality.* 1976; New York: Plenum Press.

Annells M, Koch T, Brown M. Client relevant care and quality of life: the trial of a Client Generated Index (CGI) tool for community nursing. *International Journal of Nursing Studies.* 2001; **38**(1): 9–16.

Bardelli D, Saracci R. Measuring the quality of life in cancer clinical trials: a sample of published trials. *IUCC Technical Report Series.* 1978; **36**: 75–79.

Berenholtz S, Provonost PJ. Barriers to translating evidence into practice. *Current Opinion in Critical Care.* 2003; **9**(4): 321–325.

Bergner M. Quality of life, health status and clinical research. *Medical Care.* 1989; **27**(3) (Suppl): 148–156.

Bergner M, Bobbitt RA, Carter WB, Gilson BS. The sickness impact profile: development and final revision of a health status measure. *Medical Care.* 1981; **19**(8): 787–805.

Bonomi AE, Patrick DL, Bushnell DM, Martin M. Validation of the United States' version of the World Health Organisation quality of life (WHOQOL) instrument. *Journal of Clinical Epidemiology.* 2000; **53**(1): 1–12.

Calman KC. Quality of life in cancer patients – an hypothesis. *Journal of Medical Ethics.* 1984; **10**(3): 124–127.

Carr AJ, Gibson B, Robinson PG. Measuring the quality of life: is quality of life determined by expectations or experience? *British Medical Journal.* 2001; **322**(7298): 1240–1243.

Carr AJ, Higginson IJ. Are quality of life measures patient centred? *British Medical Journal.* 2001; **322**(7298): 1357–1360.

Cohen SR, Mount MM, Tomas JJN, Mount LF. Existential well-being is an important determinant of quality of life. *Cancer.* 1996; **77**(3): 576–586.

Dalkey NC, Rourke D, Lewis R, Snyder D. *Studies in the Quality of Life.* 1972; Lexington, MA: Lexington Books, pp3–8.

Degner LF, Kristjanson LJ, Bownan D, Sloan IA, Carriere KC *et al.* Information needs and decisional preferences in women with breast cancer. *Journal of the American Medical Association.* 1997; **277**(18): 1485–1490.

Department of Health. *Equity and Excellence: liberating the NHS* (Cm7881). 2010; London: The Stationery Office. Available at: www.dh.gov.uk/en/Publicationsandstatistics/Publications/PublicationsPolicyAndGuidance/DH_117353. Last accessed 15 February 2012.

Evers G. Comments on 'The quality of life: design and evaluation of a self-assessment instrument for use with cancer patients'. *International Journal of Nursing Studies.* 2003; **40**(5): 521–523.

Fallowfield LJ. Assessment of quality of life in breast cancer. *Acta Oncologica.* 1995; **34**(5): 687–694.

Farquhar M. Definitions of quality of life: a taxonomy. *Journal of Advanced Nursing.* 1995; **22**(3):502–508.

Ferrans CE. Quality of life: conceptual issues. *Seminars in Oncology Nursing.* 1990; **6**(4): 248–254.

Ferrans CE. Development of a conceptual model for quality of life. *Scholarly Inquiry for Nursing Practice.* 1996; **10**(3): 293–304.

Guyatt GH. Measurement of health-related quality of life in heart failure. *Journal of the American College of Cardiology*. 1993; **22**(4): 185A–191A.

Haas BK. A multidisciplinary concept analysis of quality of life. *Western Journal of Nursing Research*. 1999; **21**(6): 728–742.

Hannestad BR. Errors of measurement affecting the reliability and validity of data acquired from self-assessed quality of life. *Scandinavian Journal of Caring Science*. 1990; **4**(1): 29–34.

Harrison MB, Juniper EF, Mitchell-DiCensa A. Quality of life as an outcome measure in nursing research. 'May you have a long and healthy life'. *Canadian Journal of Nursing Research*. 1996; **28**(3): 49–68.

Hickey AM, Bury G, O'Boyle CA, Bradley F, O'Kelly FD, Shannon W. A new short form individual quality of life measure (SEIQOL-DW): application in a cohort of individuals with HIV/AIDS. *British Medical Journal*. 1996; **313**(7048): 29–31.

Higginson IJ, Carr AJ. Measuring quality of life: using quality of life measures in the clinical setting. *British Medical Journal*. 2001; **322**(7297): 1297–1300.

Higginson IJ, McCarthy M. A comparison of two measures of quality of life: their sensitivity and validity for patients with advanced cancer. *Palliative Medicine*. 1994; **8**(4): 282–290.

Holmes S. A study of quality of life in Internet health chat room users. *Journal of Research in Nursing*. 2006; **11**(2): 118–129.

Holmes S, Dickerson J. The quality of life: design and evaluation of a self-assessment instrument for use with cancer patients. *International Journal of Nursing Studies*. 1987; **24**(1): 25–33.

Jacobs V. Informational needs of surgical patients following discharge. *Applied Nursing Research*. 2000; **13**(1): 12–18.

Jones D, Fayers PN, Simons J. Measuring and analysing quality of life in cancer clinical trials: a review. In: NK Aaronson and J Beckmann (eds). *The Quality of Life of Cancer Patients*. 1987; New York: Raven Press, pp41–61.

Keith KD. International quality of life: current conceptual, measurement, and implementation issues. In: LM Glidden (ed.). *International Review of Research in Mental Retardation*. 2001; San Diego, CA: Academic Press, p49.

King CR, Haberman M, Berry DL, Bush N, Butler L *et al.* Quality of life and the cancer experience: the state-of-the-knowledge. *Oncology Nursing Forum*. 1997; **24**(1): 27–41.

Koller M, Klinkhammer-Schalke M, Lorenz W. Outcome and quality of life in medicine: a conceptual framework to put quality of life research into practice. *Urologic Oncology*. 2005; **23**(3): 186–192.

Leidy NK, Coughlen C. Psychometric performance of the asthma quality of life questionnaire in a US sample. *Quality of Life Research*. 1998; **7**(2): 127–134.

Leininger M. Quality of life from a transcultural nursing perspective. *Nursing Science Quarterly*. 1994; **7**: 22–28.

Leplege A, Hunt S. The problem of quality of life in medicine. *Journal of the American Medical Association*. 1997; **278**(1): 47–50.

McCorkle R, Young K. Development of a symptom distress scale. *Cancer Nursing*. 1978; **1**(5): 373–378.

Macduff C. Respondent-generated quality of life measures: useful tools for nursing or more fool's gold? *Journal of Advanced Nursing*. 2000; **23**(2): 375–382.

Malloch K. The white lies of leadership: caring dishonesty? *Nursing Administration Quarterly*. 2001; **25**(3): 61–68.

Mandzuk LL, McMillan DE. A concept analysis of quality of life. *Journal of Orthopaedic Nursing*. 2005; **9**(1): 12–18.

Moons P, Budts W, De Geest S. Critique on the conceptualization of quality of life: a review and evaluation of different conceptual approaches. *International Journal of Nursing Studies*. 2006; **43**(7): 891–901.

National Center for Chronic Disease Prevention and Health Promotion. Health related quality of life. Available at: **www.cdc.gov/hrqol/**. Accessed 2 October 2011.

Neugarten F, Havighurst R, Tobin S. The measurement of life satisfaction. *Journal of Gerontology*. 1961; **16**: 134–143.

New Economics Foundation, National Accounts of Wellbeing. 2009; London. Also available at: **www.nationalaccountsofwellbeing.org/**. Accessed 15 October 2011.

Parse RR. Quality of life: sciencing and living the art of human becoming. *Nursing Science Quarterly*. 1994; **7**(1): 16–21.

Patrick DL, Bergner M. Measurement of health status in the 1990s. *Annual Review of Public Health*. 1990; **11**: 165–183.

Pellegrino ED. Decisions to withdraw life-sustaining treatment: a moral algorithm. *Journal of the American Medical Association*. 2000; **283**(8): 1065–1067.

Phillips JR. Quality of life research: its increasing importance. *Nursing Science Quarterly*. 1995; **8**(3): 100–101.

Plummer M, Molzahn AE. Quality of life in contemporary nursing theory: a concept analysis. *Nursing Science Quarterly*. 2009; **22**(2): 134–140.

Rothman MC, Revicki DA. Issues in the management of health status in asthma research. *Medical Care*. 1993; **31**(Suppl): MS82–MS92.

Rotstein Z, Bara Y, Noy S, Achiron A. Quality of life in multiple sclerosis: development and validation of the 'RAYS' scale and comparison with the SF-36. *International Journal for Quality in Health Care*. 2000; **12**(6): 511–517.

Schipper H, Clinch J, Powell V. Definitions and conceptual issues. In: B Spilker (ed.). *Quality of Life Assessments in Clinical Trials*. 1990; New York: Raven Press.

Scott LD, Setter-Kline K, Britton AS. The effects of nursing interventions to enhance mental health and quality of life among individuals with heart failure. *Applied Nursing Research*. 2004; **17**: 248–256.

Scott NW, Fayers PM, Aaronson NK, Bottomley A, de Graeff A *et al*. The relationship between overall quality of life and its subdimensions was influenced by culture: analysis of an international database. *Journal of Clinical Epidemiology*. 2008; **61**(8): 788–795.

Shin DC, Johnson DM. Avowed happiness as an overall assessment of the quality of life. *Social Indicators Research*. 1978; **5**(1–4): 475–492.

Skevington S. Measuring quality of life in Britain. Introducing the WHOQOL-100. *Journal of Psychosomatic Research*. 1999; **47**(5): 449–459.

Spiroch CR, Walsh D, Mazanec P, Nelson KA. Ask the patient: a semi-structured interview study of quality of life in advanced cancer. *American Journal of Hospice and Palliative Care*. 2000; **17**(4): 235–240.

Sprangers M. Quality-of-life assessment in oncology. *Acta Oncologica*. 2002; **41**(3): 229–237.

Sprangers M, Schwartz CE. Integrating response shift into health-related quality of life: a theoretical model. *Social Science and Medicine*. 1999; **48**(11): 1507–1515.

Stewart M, Brown JB, Donner A, McWhinney IR, Oates J *et al.* The impact of patient-centered care on outcomes. *Journal of Family Practice*. 2000; **49**(9): 796–804.

Thompson IE, Melia KM, Boyd KM. *Nursing Ethics*. Third edition. 2000; Singapore: Longman Publishers.

von Essen L, Sjoden P. Perceived importance of caring behaviours to Swedish psychiatric inpatients and staff, with comparisons to somatically ill samples. *Research in Nursing and Health*. 1993; **16**(4): 293–303.

Wilson JB, Cleary PD. Linking clinical variables with health-related quality of life. *Journal of the American Medical Association*. 1995; **273**(1): 59–65.

World Health Organisation Quality of Life Group (WHO). The World Health Organisation quality of life assessment (WHOQOL): position paper from the WHO. *Social Science and Medicine*. 1995; **41**(10): 347–352.

Zigmund AS, Snaith RP. The hospital anxiety and depression scale. *Acta Psychiatrica Scandinavica*. 1983; **67**(6): 361–370.

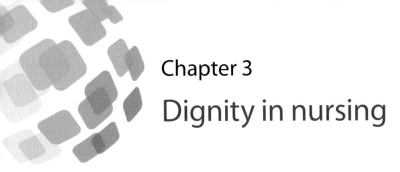

# Chapter 3

# Dignity in nursing

Despite decades of research and statements of good practice, newspaper headlines still catch my eye on trains and buses which proclaim, 'Nursing is no longer the caring profession' (*Scottish Daily Telegraph*, 30.08.2011) or 'New nurses lack caring skills' (*The Times*, 22.09.2011). Even inquiry reports state that deficiencies in 'basic nursing care as opposed to clinical errors (led) to injury or death' (Francis Report 2010 p9). And Peter Carter, Chief Executive and General Secretary of the RCN, spoke on the radio about being truly shocked by the failure of nurses 'to treat patients with the respect and dignity they deserve', this time in response to the Care Quality Commission's (CQC) first reports on dignity and nutrition for older people published in May 2011 (see Box 3.1). Surely there has been enough research to change this attitude, to acknowledge that high-quality nursing is about caring in a skilled way, making sure the basics (or rather essentials) are right and that dignified care is a central tenet of excellence in care for everyone.

This chapter reviews key research studies focused on dignity for older people, allows you glimpses of the motivations of some of the central researchers in this field and concludes by asking why the findings from these studies are still not universally implemented.

| Box 3.1 | Care Quality Commission Report on dignity and nutrition for older people press release |
|---|---|

CQC publish first of detailed reports into dignity and nutrition for older people 26 May 2011

The Care Quality Commission (CQC) today publishes the first 12 reports from an inspection programme which examines whether elderly people receive essential standards of care in 100 NHS hospitals throughout England.

The programme focuses on whether people are treated with dignity and respect, and whether they get food and drink that meet their needs. ...

These first 12 inspection reports identify three hospitals as failing to meet the essential standards required by law: Worcestershire Acute Hospitals NHS Trust, the Ipswich Hospital NHS Trust and the Royal Free Hampstead NHS Trust. Less serious concerns were identified in a further three hospitals, with the remaining six found to be meeting essential standards. All the hospitals where concerns have been identified must now tell the regulator how and when they will improve. The three hospitals failing to meet essential standards could face enforcement action by the regulator if improvements aren't made.

Whilst the reports document many examples of people being treated with respect and given personalized, attentive care, some tell a bleak story of people not being helped to eat and drink, with their care needs not assessed and their dignity not respected.

Recurring concerns relating to nutrition included:

- people not being given the assistance they needed to eat – meaning they struggled to eat and in some cases were physically unable to eat meals;
- their nutritional needs not being assessed and monitored – for example, not being weighed throughout their stay, making it impossible to determine if they were losing weight; or identified as malnourished without an action plan being put in place to address this;
- people not being given enough to drink – water left out of reach or no fluids given for long periods of time. In one case, a member of clinical staff described having to prescribe water on medicine charts to ensure patients got enough to drink.

Recurring concerns around dignity and respect included:

- people not involved in their own care – their treatment not explained to them; being told what would happen to them without consent being sought or concerns addressed; staff addressing patients' relatives rather than the patient themselves;
- staff not treating people in a respectful way – spooning food into people's mouths from above without engaging with them; discussing personal patient information in open areas;
- staff speaking to people in a condescending or dismissive way. One man told us that staff 'talk to me as if I'm daft'.

However, inspection teams also observed examples of excellent care delivered by nurses and other healthcare staff who took the time to explain every aspect of a patient's care to them in a way they could understand, interacted with each patient as an individual, spoke to them with respect and ensured their dignity was maintained. And in many hospitals, nutrition and hydration were recognized as an important part of the patient's recovery, and real efforts were made to ensure that people got meals they enjoyed in a pleasant environment – and the help they needed to eat it. One patient told us: 'I cannot praise them enough. I am made to feel that I am the most important person.'

**www.cqc.org.uk//newsandevents/pressreleases.cfm?cit_
id=37384&FAArea1=customWidgets.content_view_1&usecache=false**

# The research story so far

While dignified care can sometimes be hard to achieve, for instance in emergency situations, promoting and maintaining dignity are vital to the delivery of high-quality, individualized care. This belief forms the bedrock of nursing: it is a fundamental guiding principle of practice based on common sense rather than on research findings – maintaining someone's dignity is simply the right thing to do. However, over the past 20 years, evidence, primarily in the form of reports on the quality of services, has shown that some nurses and health and social care professionals have not paid enough attention to this fundamental element of care, and patients from a variety of specialities (e.g. services for people with learning disabilities, with mental health problems, for older people) have experienced undignified care. This has led not only to professional recriminations and outrage from families and friends but also to a burgeoning of research attention focused on why this might have happened. The following research teams have been at the forefront of work in this area.

Win Tadd (see Box 3.2) started researching dignity across Europe at the start of this millennium – she and her colleagues were keen to find out what dignity really meant to people and what would make a difference to their feelings of dignity (Bayer *et al* 2005). They found that the experience of dignity depended on several things: being recognized as an equal human being, being able to maintain personal identity and self-respect, being treated with respect by others and being able to exercise control even if you were reliant on others for help. In addition, they found that the 1,400 older people and health and social care professionals in their study felt that dignity could be compromised by illness, increased dependence (especially for those who were very old) and reduced social and economic resources.

| Box 3.2 | Win Tadd |
| --- | --- |

My research into dignity was fired by the *Observer* campaign in 1997 when the journalist Martin Bright wrote a series of moving accounts of the treatment his 88-year-old grandmother received when she was admitted to hospital following a stroke. Many older people and their relatives added their voices to this campaign and reading the harrowing accounts which echoed some of my own experiences when gathering data for my own PhD, I knew this was an area to which I wanted to contribute.

The government responded by commissioning an independent report from the Health Advisory Service, *Not Because They Are Old* (Health Advisory Service (HAS) 1999), which identified poor standards of care and a lack of dignity in the care of older people on acute wards. After contacting the researchers I discovered that this study would not define what either dignity or dignified care meant in relation to older people. In 1999 I was fortunate to receive funding from the European Commission to explore dignity in the lives of older people and have continued to work in this area for the past 12 years.

More recently, Win Tadd and her colleagues completed a study funded by the National Institute for Health Research Service Delivery and Organisation programme (NIHR-SDO) to investigate dignity in acute wards in four hospitals in England and Wales through ethnography. (Ethnographies use primarily interviews, observations and documentary analysis to collect information.) Four important themes emerged from their work (see Box 3.3); each can be used to point towards improvements in the delivery and management of care.

---

**Box 3.3    Tadd *et al's* (2011 pp9–11) themes**

**'Whose Interests Matter?'**

This theme explored the conflict of interest between the priorities of the Trust, the staff and the patients. The findings emphasize the importance of, for instance, things that can be measured, adherence to protocols of care, high bed occupancy meaning that older people were frequently moved around the hospital. Short staffing meant strict working protocols had to be adhered to and continuity of care, which promotes dignity, was often compromised.

**'Right Place – Wrong Patient'**

Within this theme staff expressed the view that the acute hospital was not the right place for older people to be cared in. The mismatch between place and patient and the resultant barriers to delivering dignified care centred on the poorly designed environments that older people were nursed in where staff, whilst doing their best, were often poorly educated and skilled in the care of older people. Additionally, the organizational goals of the Trusts were associated with quick turnover and measurable targets rather than the longer-term individualized care required by some older patients.

**'Seeing the Person'**

This theme emphasized the invisibility of older people whilst they were patients in hospital. It also stressed how being patronizing jeopardized respectful communication – this was made worse when people were referred to as a task or a number, or were ignored. Care was task-centred and often in response to patients' requests for care, making them feel dependent on staff and minimizing their sense of control over themselves and their environment. Often fundamental care (privacy, nutrition, using the toilet, washing and dressing, and being informed) was deficient, thereby leading to a feeling of loss of identity and compromised dignity. Patients were often moved within or between wards, which resulted in disorientation and a view that they should not be in an acute ward anyway. Additionally, the researchers noted the importance of staff being treated themselves with dignity by their peers, superiors and managers – failure to do this resulted in demoralization and the creation of disrespectful working environments.

**'Influences on Dignified Care'**

Key barriers and enablers of dignified care emerged from the three themes above and were listed in relation to the environment, the knowledge and skills of staff and the organizational processes of the Trusts. These will be explored in more depth at the end of this chapter.

Alongside Win Tadd's decade of work, Julienne Meyer (see Box 3.4) and her team of researchers at City University have been focusing on care in the private and voluntary sectors.

| Box 3.4 | Julienne Meyer |
|---|---|

As an action researcher, I have always been interested in doing research 'with' and 'for' people, rather than 'on' them. To me, the methodological approach offers a more dignified way of conducting research – working in partnership with those in practice, listening to the perspectives of all key stakeholders within a whole system and exploring the lessons learnt (process and outcomes) from attempts to improve practice within everyday contexts.

More recently, I have become committed to doing this in a more appreciative way. I don't understand why researchers tend to focus on problems and then blame practitioners for what they get wrong. Why not take a more positive approach by focusing on 'what people want' and 'what works'? It is my belief that this positive relational approach, which values and respects not only the needs of service users but also the needs of informal carers and service providers, is what will ultimately deliver dignified care.

It is for this reason that promoting positive 'relationships' is core to all that I do. For instance, it is central to 'Everybody Matters: Sustaining Dignity in Care' in acute care (**www.city.ac.uk/dignityincare**) and to 'My Home Life', a UK-wide initiative to promote quality of life in care homes (**www.myhomelife.org.uk**).

Key messages from this work about dignity include 'See who I am!', 'Involve me!' and 'Connect with me!', together with the need to 'Stop, Look, Listen and Appreciate!' I believe these messages are important to all those in practice, research and education.

The largest of their projects has also focused on older people and is known as the *My Home Life* (MHL) project. This project, run in conjunction with Age UK and the Joseph Rowntree Foundation, grew from a review of best practice carried out by the National Care Homes Research and Development Forum (NCHR&D Forum). The review involved 60 researchers working in partnership with care home practitioners, independent advisors and voluntary groups to examine evidence on the quality of life of older people in care homes. The review helped to identify eight best practice themes (see Box 3.5) (Help the Aged 2007), all of which impact on dignity. Since its inception the MHL project has spawned 'a growing social movement to improve practice in care homes' (Meyer 2011), fundamentally grounded in the importance of establishing dignified relationships.

Closer to home, I'm also involved in a project with Christina Victor at Brunel University, which focuses on dignity, but rather than focusing on patients and their relatives we're concentrating on front-line and managerial staff. The idea behind the project complements some of Win Tadd's and Julienne Meyer's findings, which suggest that the culture within which care is delivered relies on the way staff feel about the maintenance

---

**Box 3.5**    *My* **Home Life best practice themes** *(my comments in italics)*

Managing transitions. (*Although focused on transitions into nursing or care homes, it is important to remember that transition to hospital can also cause anxiety and awkwardness.*)

Maintaining identity.

Creating community. (*For those of you thinking about the hospital environment this theme is important to consider when nursing people with extended admissions. Creating community is also an important aspect for staff – they, too, need to feel that they work in a community where they are respected and can develop and sustain excellence in care.*)

Sharing decision making.

Improving health and healthcare.

Supporting good end-of-life.

Keeping the workforce fit for purpose.

Promoting a positive culture (*which values dignity as particularly important for staff and patients*).

**http://myhomelifemovement.org/best-practice-themes/**

---

**Box 3.6**    **Deborah Cairns**

My name is Deborah Cairns and I'm a researcher working on a project which aims to explore how dignified care for older people is understood and delivered by the health and social care workforce and how organizational structures and policies can promote and facilitate, or hinder, the delivery of dignified care.

I wanted to work on this project as I'm very passionate about dignified care. Professionally, I have cared for older vulnerable adults and, personally, I have had loved ones who have spent time in hospital, and I believe that dignity is the foundation of any care.

My current role is really exciting because I have the opportunity to promote dignified care, share important findings with different professionals and hopefully make changes for the better.

---

of their own dignity at work. We are exploring this through a survey and also trying to establish the challenges staff face in providing dignified care through a series of story-telling interviews. You can read in Box 3.6 what it's like for Deborah Cairns to be working as a researcher on this project.

## What influences dignified care?

As a result of their study, Win Tadd's research team developed a comprehensive list of environmental barriers, knowledge and skills deficits and organizational processes that impinge on dignity in acute wards (Tadd *et al* 2011 pp4–5); they have also highlighted several enablers of dignified care. The barriers include:

- disorientating physical environments in acute wards;
- few opportunities for patients to interact with other people in community spaces or engage in stimulating activities, resulting in boredom and dejection;
- patients being given insufficient information about ward routines and staff;
- staff having insufficient knowledge of the needs of people with dementia;
- frequent movement of older patients within and between wards;
- an organizational view that older people should not be being cared for on acute wards.

Some enablers of dignified care are listed below:

- examples of environments which were well suited to the needs of older patients with careful use of signage, colour, communal areas, boards giving relevant and readable information;
- adequate space between beds to promote privacy;
- gender-specific facilities for washing as well as toilets;
- staff appraisal mechanisms that encouraged reflection on practice and took account of patient experiences;
- courteous and respectful communication;
- patient-centred practice and organizational management;
- social activities that are relevant to different age groups;
- collaborative team working;
- respectful attitudes of staff to patients and colleagues.

In addition to these studies focused specifically on older people, Lesley Baillie's (2009) research has concentrated on understanding what dignity (or its absence) means to all age groups of people receiving acute care in hospitals. As you can see in Box 3.7, she first got interested as a result of a personal experience. Her work also emphasizes the important role that staff play in promoting dignity through maintaining comfort, encouraging patients to remain in control of their decisions and care, and ensuring that people (staff and patients) feel valued. Baillie's work accentuates the intrinsic relationship between dignity and respect and the importance of mutual respect between patients and their carers in constructing dignified care and environments.

| Box 3.7 | Lesley Baillie |
|---|---|

As a nurse, and a teacher of nurses, I often spoke of 'dignity' when talking about patient care and I assumed that I knew what dignity meant. However, a personal experience led me to question the concept more deeply.

My mother was seriously ill in hospital and one evening she said to me, with despair, 'I've lost all my dignity now. There's none left.' I felt perplexed: my mother was in a side room and staff seemed respectful. A few days later she died and in the months following, I pondered what she'd said. I started to question: what is dignity and could anything have restored her dignity? This led me to carry out my research study about patient dignity in hospital.

---

**Exercise 3.1  Baillie's case study**

Read Lesley Baillie's (2009) paper and compare her findings with your experiences of nursing people requiring acute medical or surgical care.

Use Baillie's case study as a trigger to help you to consider why dignity, in its broadest sense, is still difficult to implement. Your ideas might also include some of the barriers identified by Tadd *et al* (2011).

Once you have jotted down your ideas, consider what might stop the findings from these studies being implemented and what might help them to be. You will read more about the implementation of research in the later chapters of this book.

---

This chapter has summarized key contemporary research studies exploring dignity associated with nursing in the UK. Having research available, as you have seen here and will see throughout this book, is not the whole story – nurses need to implement the best research into practice to improve the quality of care delivered to patients and their carers/families as well as their quality of life.

## ◼ Further reading

Milika RM, Baillie L (eds). *Dignity in Healthcare: A practical approach*. 2011; Oxford: Radcliffe Publishing Ltd. This book provides an evidence-based overview of dignity across the spectrum of care.

Nolan M, Brown J, Davies S, Nolan J, Keady J. The Senses Framework: Improving care for older people through a relationship-centred approach. *Getting Research into Practice (GRiP) Report No 2*. 2006; University of Sheffield. Available at: http://shura.shu. ac.uk/280/1/PDF_Senses_Framework_Report.pdf. This research report details an approach to providing dignified person-centred care to older people.

## ◼ References

Baillie L. Patient dignity in an acute hospital setting: a case study. *International Journal of Nursing Studies*. 2009; **46**(1): 23–36.

Bayer A, Tadd W, Krajcik S. Dignity: the voice of older people. *Quality in Ageing*. 2005; **6**(1): 22–29.

Francis R. *Independent inquiry into care provided by Mid Staffordshire NHS Foundation Trust, January 2005–March 2009*. 2010; London: Department of Health.

Health Advisory Service (HAS). *Not Because They Are Old: An independent inquiry into the care of older people on acute wards in general hospitals.* 1999; London: The Stationery Office.

Help the Aged. *My Home Life: Quality of life in care homes: A review of the literature.* 2007; London: Help the Aged. Available at: http://myhomelifemovement.org/downloads/mhl_review.pdf.

Meyer J. Review: Nursing home culture, teamwork and culture change. *Journal of Research in Nursing.* 2011; **16**(1): 51–52.

Milika R, Baillie L (eds). *Dignity in Healthcare: A practical approach.* 2011; Oxford: Radcliffe Publishing Ltd.

Nolan M, Brown J, Davies S, Nolan J, Keady J. The Senses Framework: improving care for older people through a relationship-centred approach. *Getting Research into Practice (GRiP) Report No 2.* 2006; University of Sheffield.

Tadd W, Hillman A, Calnan S *et al. Dignity in Practice: An exploration of the care of older adults in acute NHS Trusts.* 2011; Southampton: NIHR-SDO.

# Chapter 4

# Pressure ulcers: prevention and care

## ▪ Introduction

The incidence and prevalence of pressure ulcers are anecdotally and empirically linked to nursing care. Griffiths *et al* (2008) in their search for markers which could be used to measure nursing's contributions to patient care found several indicators, the most frequently identified being the occurrence of pressure ulcers. Over the last two decades in the UK alone several million pounds have been spent on research focusing on pressure ulcer prevention and care in an attempt to reduce the significant financial burden for health and social care providers and the personal burden for patients and their families associated with this condition.

---

**Exercise 4.1   Thinking about the cost of pressure ulcers**

To get a better idea of the financial cost of different grades of pressure ulcers look at the DH (2010) Pressure Ulcer Productivity Calculator.

**www.dh.gov.uk/en/Publicationsandstatistics/Publications/
PublicationsPolicyAndGuidance/DH_116669**

---

As a consequence of their financial and personal impact, pressure ulcers have been the subject of much research. While this shows the priority that research funders have placed on this area of practice, it also means that there is a large quantity of research to sift through before finding the key studies of immediate relevance to care. Knowing where to start in such circumstances is a challenge. As a result, this chapter starts the search for research not with a literature review but by looking at the key guidelines produced by the National Institute for Health and Clinical Excellence (NICE) and the Royal College of Nursing (RCN). These are research-led guidelines and, as such, are based on the most up-to-date, rigorous and clinically relevant research.

# ■ The guidelines

My search started at the website for the National Clinical Guideline Centre (www.ncgc. ac.uk/), a multi-disciplinary health services research team funded by NICE to produce evidence-based clinical practice guidelines. Here I found two guidelines originally published by NICE – one on pressure ulcer management (published in 2005) and the other on risk assessment and pressure-relieving devices (published in 2003). A further foray into the website confirmed that both guidelines were still available but were both shortly to be updated and replaced.

---

### Exercise 4.2  Keeping up to date

Go to the National Clinical Guideline Centre's website (**www.ncgc.ac.uk/**) and check whether the new guidelines have been published. Check when they are due for review (a date will be shown) and make a note to check them again during this period of time in order to identify any necessary changes to practice.

Another good way to keep up to date with new research is to review regularly the contents of the journal *Evidence-Based Nursing*. In the July 2011 issue (volume 14, number 3) you will find a useful commentary by Beeckman and Vanderwee (2011: 79–80) on research focused on wheelchair cushions for the prevention of pressure ulcers.

---

These publications gave me some useful background information.

- First, both guidelines (2003 and 2005) were developed by the Royal College of Nursing with other key stakeholders and adopted by NICE.
- Second, they should be read in conjunction with each other.
- Third, there are three key research groups focusing on pressure ulcer research related to nursing care. One at the University of Manchester under the direction of Nicky Cullum (www.nursing.manchester.ac.uk); another at Leeds University (www.healthcare.leeds.ac.uk/research/symptom-management-and-long-term-conditions/); and the last at the University of Wales, College of Medicine (www. whru.co.uk/cnt/homeh.asp). It is always useful to locate key researcher groups in specific clinical areas so that you can follow their work and look out for their next publications.
- Fourth, there is a Cochrane Wounds Group. You can find out more about this group at http://wounds.cochrane.org/.
- Finally, there is a large amount of research out there and the only way for any practitioner to make sense of it all is to look for work (either guidelines or systematic reviews) that has brought together all the relevant research, appraised it and synthesized it into a list of research-based recommendations.

## What the guidelines tell us

Both of these guidelines make specific recommendations for practice based on the research available, and where there has been no research undertaken, a review of best practice. The guidelines have been rigorously constructed and practitioners can rely on them (albeit with one proviso – they are both currently being updated). The key recommendations from both sets of guidelines can be seen in Table 4.1.

**Table 4.1**  What the guidelines tell us (RCN 2003; 2005)

| The use of pressure-relieving devices (beds, mattresses and overlays) for the prevention of pressure ulcers in primary and secondary care (RCN 2003 pp10–11) | The management of pressure ulcers in primary and secondary care (RCN 2005 pp22–23) |
|---|---|
| Decisions about which pressure-relieving device to use should be based on cost considerations and an overall assessment of the individual. Holistic assessment should include all of the following points, and should not be based solely on scores from risk assessment scales:<br><br>• identified levels of risk;<br><br>• skin assessment;<br><br>• comfort;<br><br>• general health state;<br><br>• lifestyle and abilities;<br><br>• critical care needs;<br><br>• acceptability of the proposed pressure-relieving equipment to the patient and/or carer.<br><br>All individuals assessed as being vulnerable to pressure ulcers should, as a minimum provision, be placed on a high-specification foam mattress with pressure-relieving properties.<br><br>Although there is no research evidence that high-tech pressure-relieving mattresses and overlays are more effective than high-specification – low-tech – foam mattresses and overlays, professional consensus recommends that consideration should be given to the use of alternating pressure or other high-tech pressure-relieving systems: | The following recommendations have been identified as priorities for implementation.<br><br>Record the pressure ulcer grade using the European Pressure Ulcer Advisory Panel Classification System.<br><br>All pressure ulcers graded 2 and above should be documented as a local clinical incident.<br><br>Patients with pressure ulcers should receive an initial and ongoing pressure ulcer assessment. Where a cause is identified, strategies should be implemented to remove/reduce these. Ulcer assessment should include:<br><br>• cause of ulcer;<br><br>• site/location;<br><br>• dimensions of ulcer;<br><br>• stage or grade;<br><br>• exudate amount and type;<br><br>• local signs of infection;<br><br>• pain;<br><br>• wound appearance;<br><br>• surrounding skin;<br><br>• undermining/tracking (sinus or fistula);<br><br>• odour; and<br><br>• involvement of clinical experts – e.g. tissue viability nurse. |

*continued* ➤

| The use of pressure-relieving devices (beds, mattresses and overlays) for the prevention of pressure ulcers in primary and secondary care (RCN 2003 pp10–11) | The management of pressure ulcers in primary and secondary care (RCN 2005 pp22–23) |
|---|---|
| • as a first-line preventative strategy for people at elevated risk, as identified by holistic assessment;<br><br>• when the individual's previous history of pressure ulcer prevention and/or clinical condition indicates that they are best cared for on a high-tech device;<br><br>• when a low-tech device has failed.<br><br>All individuals undergoing surgery and assessed as being vulnerable to pressure ulcers should, as a minimum provision, be placed on either a high-specification foam theatre mattress or other pressure-relieving surface.<br><br>The provision of pressure-relieving devices needs a 24-hour approach. It should include consideration of all surfaces used by the patient.<br><br>Support surface and positioning needs should be assessed and reviewed regularly and determined by the results of skin inspection, patient comfort, ability and general state. Thus repositioning should occur when individuals are on pressure-relieving devices.<br><br>The management of a patient in a sitting position is also important. Even with appropriate pressure relief, it may be necessary to restrict sitting time to less than two hours until the condition of an individual with an elevated risk changes.<br><br>A pressure ulcer reduction strategy should incorporate a coordinated approach to the acquisition, allocation and management of pressure-relieving equipment. The time elapsing between assessment and use of the device should be specified in this strategy.<br><br>All healthcare professionals should be educated about:<br><br>• pressure ulcer risk assessment and prevention;<br><br>• selection, use and maintenance of pressure-relieving devices;<br><br>• patient education and information-giving. | This should be supported by tracings and/or photography (calibrated with a ruler).<br><br>Patients with pressure ulcers should have access to pressure-relieving support surfaces and strategies – for example, mattresses and cushions – 24 hours a day, and this applies to all support surfaces.<br><br>All individuals assessed as having a grade 1–2 pressure ulcer should, as a minimum provision, be placed on a high-specification foam mattress or cushion with pressure-reducing properties combined with very close observation of skin changes, and a documented positioning and repositioning regime.<br><br>If there is any perceived or actual deterioration of affected areas or further pressure ulcer development, an alternating pressure (AP) (replacement or overlay) or sophisticated continuous low pressure (CLP) system – for example low air loss, air fluidised, air flotation, viscous fluid – should be used. (NB: For individuals requiring bed rails, AP overlay mattresses should be placed on a reduced-depth foam mattress to maintain their safety.)<br><br>Depending on the location of the ulcer, individuals assessed as having grade 3–4 pressure ulcers – including intact eschar where depth, and therefore grade, cannot be assessed – should, as a minimum provision, be placed on an alternating pressure mattress (replacement or overlay) or sophisticated continuous low pressure system – for example low air loss, air fluidised, viscous fluid.<br><br>*continued* ➤ |

| The use of pressure-relieving devices (beds, mattresses and overlays) for the prevention of pressure ulcers in primary and secondary care (RCN 2003 pp10–11) | The management of pressure ulcers in primary and secondary care (RCN 2005 pp22–23) |
| --- | --- |
| Individuals vulnerable to or at elevated risk of developing pressure ulcers, and their carers, should be informed verbally and in writing about: <ul><li>the prevention of pressure ulcers using pressure-relieving strategies;</li><li>the use and maintenance of pressure-relieving devices;</li><li>where they can seek further advice and assistance.</li></ul> | If alternating pressure equipment is required, the first choice should be an overlay system, unless other circumstances such as patient weight or patient safety indicate the need for a replacement system. <br><br> Create the optimum wound healing environment by using modern dressings – for example hydrocolloids, hydrogels, hydrofibres, foams, films, alginates, soft silicones – in preference to basic dressing types – for example gauze, paraffin gauze and simple dressing pads. |

Each of the recommendations is graded A–D in the original documents depending on the research evidence available to support the statement (A being the strongest), i.e. the type of research design and the rigour with which the study was carried out (you will read more about this later in the book). Go to these documents and see for yourself how this is done.

The research evidence underpinning these guidelines came from a variety of designs, including:

- prospective cohort studies;
- surveys;
- randomized controlled trials;
- economic evaluations.

These types of research design are the most rigorous and, therefore, rightly used to underpin clinical guidelines. As you read Chapters 5 and 6 you will become more familiar with these designs and what they have to offer. Rarely were qualitative studies used in formulating the guidelines – this means that readers are left asking questions about the experiences of patients with pressure ulcers and how these impact on their quality of life. Exercise 4.3 will give you an idea about the experiences of people living with pressure ulcers.

---

**Exercise 4.3  Finding out more about living with pressure ulcers**

You might find it useful to look for research which specifically addresses this aspect of pressure ulcers in order to enhance your practice. Some research studies that you will find useful are:

Langemo *et al*. The lived experience of having a pressure ulcer: a qualitative analysis. *Advances in Skin and Wound Care*. 2000; **13**(5): 225–235.

Spilsbury *et al*. Pressure ulcers and their treatment and effects on quality of life: hospital inpatient perspectives. *Journal of Advanced Nursing*. 2007; **57**(5): 494–504.

Read these papers and consider how knowledge of the findings from these studies will make your practice better.

---

# ■ Is anything else needed?

Once the guidelines and underpinning research are located they need to be integrated into practice. This, as you can see from the clip from the Care Quality Commission's (CQC) report on North Devon District Hospital (Box 4.1), will rely not only on the appropriate research being found and used but also on accurate documentation, skilled communication and team work. Using research without these accompanying essentials of good practice is not going to be effective enough.

| Box 4.1 | Improvements needed |
|---|---|

Care Quality Commission tells North Devon District Hospital to improve wound care: 25 August 2011

The Care Quality Commission has told Northern Devon Healthcare NHS Trust that it must improve its systems for managing wound care and for dealing with patients who are at risk of developing pressure sores.

Inspectors who visited North Devon District Hospital in Barnstaple found that care plans and other patient records were not always completed. While they did not find individual cases of poor care, they did find a failure to fully assess and plan all aspects of patient care, which could mean that some people might not get the care they needed.

The inspection focused on the hospital's current compliance in four related areas:

- how pressure area care is managed;
- how well the hospital works with patients with complex needs or with communication difficulties;
- consent and assessing mental capacity for patients;
- meeting nutritional and hydration needs.

Inspectors spent three days at the hospital in July, meeting patients and staff, checking records and visiting medical and surgical wards. They found that the Trust was compliant with three of the four standards which were reviewed.

## Respecting and involving people

Inspectors found that people's independence, privacy and dignity were respected and they were able to make informed choices and express their views. Improvements were needed to ensure that, where possible, individuals' needs and preferences were fully documented. For people with dementia this includes consulting with their carers and ensuring they are always treated with dignity and respect.

## Consent to care and treatment

The report concludes that there were processes to ensure that people, including those who lacked capacity, could give informed consent to their care and treatment. While the hospital met the requirements of the Mental Capacity Act, some improvements were needed to ensure consent was fully documented for all areas of treatment and care, such as the use of bed rails.

## Meeting nutritional needs

Records showed that risk assessments were recorded properly, and where needed, referrals were made to dieticians and speech and language therapists for swallowing assessments. Assessments had been made and reviewed in respect of people who may be at risk of malnourishment. Inspectors concluded that people's dietary and nutritional needs were being met.

## Care and welfare of patients

The Trust was not compliant with this standard. Inspectors found examples where patients' care plans, wound care plans and pressure area assessments were not recorded properly. They found eight examples of wound care plans where the records were unclear about when treatment started or whether improvements were being properly monitored. Inspectors concluded that people were at risk of receiving inappropriate care because care plans and monitoring records were incomplete. Failure to fully assess and plan the delivery of all aspects of care and treatment meant that their needs might not be met properly.

Ian Biggs, Regional Director of CQC in the South West, said that the Trust must now provide its plans to show how it will achieve full compliance. He said: 'In a busy hospital, good patient records are essential. Doctors and nurses depend on them to ensure that their patients are getting the right care throughout the day and night, when shifts change and different staff come on duty or take over responsibility for a particular person's care. Patients we met on the wards had no complaints about their care, although we have identified some key areas of concern, mainly around pressure damage and wound care, where lack of assessment and care planning could place people at risk.'

**www.cqc.org.uk/newsandevents/newsstories.cfm?FaArea1=customwidgets. content_view_1&cit_id=37562**

Both of the RCN guidelines provide criteria against which to audit following their implementation. Having these specific criteria makes it much easier when you want to measure any improvement in care. You can see an excerpt from the audit criteria created to accompany the guidelines on the management of pressure ulcers in primary and secondary care (RCN 2005) in Table 4.2; these criteria relate to documentation as well as to direct patient care.

**Table 4.2**  Audit criteria related to the guideline on the management of pressure ulcers in primary and secondary care (RCN 2005 p210)

| Criterion | Exception | Definition of terms |
|---|---|---|
| 1. The individual's plan of care contains a classification/grade for all pressure ulcers using the European Pressure Ulcer Advisory Panel (EPUAP) classification system. | None | The grade of ulcers should be clearly documented in the plan of care to be available to the inter-disciplinary team. Pressure ulcers should be given a grade of 1–4. Pressure ulcers should not be reverse graded in that a healing grade 4 pressure ulcer should be described as such and not as a grade 3 pressure ulcer. |
| 2. A pressure ulcer that is identified as a grade 2 or above is documented as a clinical incident. | None | The reporting should follow Trust procedure for reporting of clinical incidents. |
| 3. Individuals with pressure ulcers have their ulcer assessed initially (within six hours) and the assessment is ongoing. The assessment is supported by tracings and/or a photograph of the ulcer. | None | The ulcer is assessed for cause, site/location, dimensions, stage/grade, exudates (amount and type), local signs of infection, pain, wound appearance, appearance of surrounding skin, undermining/tracking (sinus or fistula), and odour. Clinical experts are involved as appropriate – e.g. tissue viability nurse. |
| 4. Individuals with pressure ulcers have access to appropriate pressure-relieving support surfaces or strategies throughout a 24-hour period. This includes all surfaces used by the individual, including mattresses and cushions. | None | Support surfaces include all surfaces used by an individual, which will include mattresses for beds (including theatre trolleys), and cushions for chairs and wheelchairs. Strategies include the use of repositioning to minimize prolonged pressure on the body. |

# Conclusion

Pressure ulcers can have a considerable negative impact on the quality of life of patients and their carers; they also take up a high proportion of health and social care providers' budgets and nursing time. Ensuring that pressure ulcer care, preventative or curative, is therefore based on the best research available is important. However, finding the best research can be challenging for every practitioner. This chapter has shown you how, when there is a plethora of research, to seek out guidelines which have, during their development, already sifted through and found the best research on which to base practice. Sometimes, however, these guidelines do not include valuable research about patients' experiences. If this is the case you need to search for rigorous qualitative research to complete your knowledge and thereby inform your practice.

Following national guidelines alone is not good enough – you need to adapt them to fit the local context within which you are working and then audit them regularly to ensure that their impact and usefulness are evaluated in practice.

## References

Beeckman D, Vanderwee K. Skin protection wheelchair cushions for older nursing home residents reduce 6 month incidence of ischial tuberosity pressure ulcers compared with segmented foam cushions. *Evidence-Based Nursing.* 2011; **14**(3): 79–80.

Griffiths P with Jones S, Maben J, Murrells T. *State of the Art Metrics for Nursing: A rapid appraisal.* 2008; London: National Nursing Research Unit, King's College London.

Langemo D, Melland H, Hanson D, Olson B, Hunter S. The lived experience of having a pressure ulcer: a qualitative analysis. *Advances in Skin and Wound Care.* 2000; **13**(5): 225–235.

Royal College of Nursing. *The Use of Pressure-relieving Devices (Beds, Mattresses and Overlays) for the Prevention of Pressure Ulcers in Primary and Secondary Care.* 2003; London: NICE.

Royal College of Nursing. *The Management of Pressure Ulcers in Primary and Secondary Care.* 2005; London: NICE.

Spilsbury K, Nelson A, Cullum N, Iglesias C, Nixon J, Mason S. Pressure ulcers and their treatment and effects on quality of life: hospital inpatient perspectives. *Journal of Advanced Nursing.* 2007; **57**(5): 494–504.

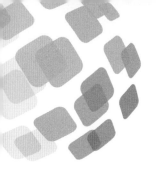

# Chapter 5

# Asking worthwhile questions for practice

## ■ Introduction

No practising nurse can justifiably doubt the value of research to the development and implementation of effective nursing care. But, in order to ensure that relevant and usable research findings are generated, researchers must first ask the right research question (no matter how large or small the research project). Getting that question right is not a simple task. This chapter describes a step-by-step, reflective approach to asking worthwhile questions that may help.

## ■ Selecting a research(able) problem

The first and most challenging part of any research project is selecting a researchable problem. This structures the research question(s) and guides the subsequent choice of the research design, the methods of data collection and analysis, and also the approaches to be used in dissemination and implementation of research findings. Essentially, the problem selected needs to be one that will make a difference to practice and, as such, one that other people – both practitioners (users of your findings) and funders – will think is important enough to support. Finding the right problem is therefore central to the success of any research project and needs careful attention.

Once, selecting areas for research was seen as the sole responsibility of researchers and funding bodies; now, however, greater emphasis is being placed on involving the people who will use the research (practitioners and service users) in the selection of areas that need researching. For the last decade the importance of public involvement in health and social care research has been championed by a national advisory group called

INVOLVE. This group aims to work 'towards creating the research community of the future which will be broader, more inclusive and more representative of the population as a whole' and so doing, they hope to 'ensure that the entire research process is focused on what is important to people and is therefore more relevant and acceptable to the users of services' (**www.invo.org.uk/**). For more information see Box 5.1 and visit the INVOLVE website.

---

**Box 5.1    INVOLVE's purpose (www.invo.org.uk/)**

INVOLVE was established to promote public involvement in research, in order to improve the way that research is prioritized, commissioned, undertaken, communicated and used. We believe that the active involvement of the public in the research process leads to research that is more relevant to people and is more likely to be used. Research which reflects the needs and views of the public is more likely to produce results that can be used to improve practice in health and social care.

We use the term 'public' to include:

- patients and potential patients;
- people who use health and social services;
- informal carers;
- parents/guardians;
- disabled people;
- members of the public who are potential recipients of health promotion programmes, public health programmes and social service interventions;
- groups asking for research because they believe they have been exposed to potentially harmful substances or products (e.g. pesticides or asbestos);
- organizations that represent people who use services.

The term 'the public' also embraces the rich diversity of people in our multicultural society, whether defined by age, colour, race, ethnicity or nationality, disability, gender or sexuality, who may have different needs and concerns. These need to be taken into account in our policies, procedures and practices.

By 'involvement' we mean: an active partnership between the public and researchers in the research process, rather than the use of people as the 'subjects' of research. Active involvement may take the form of consultation, collaboration or user control. Many people define public involvement in research as doing research 'with' or 'by' the public, rather than 'to', 'about' or 'for' the public. This would include, for example, public involvement in advising on a research project, assisting in the design of a project, or in carrying out the research.

Why not encourage some people you know to get involved? You will find useful information at the 'People in Research' website (**www.peopleinresearch.org/**). Or, if you're considering embarking on a research project, think about how you might get members of the public involved in your project. (The James Lind Alliance has developed a democratic consensus-reaching technique for creating research questions which can be used by healthcare professionals and patients. Have a look at the website (**www. lindalliance.org/**) or read Lloyd and White's (2011) paper.)

INVOLVE is not alone in trying to encourage non-researchers to participate in the design of research or the identification of problems that need research – all of the National Institute for Health Research (NIHR) funded programmes (see Box 5.2) do this, too (see Box 5.3).

| Box 5.2 | National Institute for Health Research (NIHR) programmes |
|---|---|

Set up by the Department of Health in England, the NIHR aims to improve the health and wealth of the nation through research. NIHR does this by 'commissioning leading-edge scientific research focused on improving quality and patient outcomes, and supporting decisions about service investment and disinvestment. It plays a critical role in the development of better approaches which lead to improved health outcomes' (**www.nihr. ac.uk/files/pdfs/Briefing%20documents/1.1%20The%20National%20 Institute%20for%20Health%20Research.pdf**).

In order to do this, NIHR funds various research projects spanning a range of topics from clinical problems to service delivery. These are clustered under a number of funding programmes, with the best known being:

The **Research for Patient Benefit** (RfPB) programme, which aims to produce  high-quality research for the benefit of users of the NHS in England (**www.ccf.nihr.ac.uk/RfPB/**).

The **Health Technology Assessment** (HTA) programme, which funds research to ensure that healthcare professionals, NHS managers and the public and patients have the best and latest information on the costs, effectiveness and impact of developments in health technology (**www.hta.ac.uk/**).

The **Health Services and Delivery Research** (HS&DR) programme, which focuses on research into the quality, appropriateness, effectiveness, equity and patient experience of health services as well as evaluating models of service organization, delivery and interventions, which have the potential to improve service effectiveness, efficiency and productivity (**www.netscc.ac.uk/hsdr/**).

The **Public Health Research** (PHR) programme, which funds research to provide new knowledge on the benefits, costs, acceptability and wider effect of non-NHS interventions, e.g. prevention of obesity in children and speed humps for the prevention of road traffic accidents (**www.phr.ac.uk/**).

Visit the NIHR website at **www.nihr.ac.uk/** to keep up to date.

| Box 5.3 | National Institute for Health Research statement on involvement |
|---|---|

Involving patients and members of the public in research can lead to better research, clearer outcomes, and faster uptake of new evidence.

The NIHR encourages patients and the public to be actively involved in all NIHR-funded health and social care research, to:

- set research priorities;
- identify the important questions that health and social care research needs to answer;
- give their views on research proposals alongside clinicians, methodologists, scientists, and public health and other professionals;
- help assess proposals for funding;
- take part in clinical trials and other health and social care research studies, not just as subjects but as active partners in the research process;
- publicise the results.

**www.nihr.ac.uk/awareness/Pages/default.aspx**

In addition to this, practitioners are invited to contribute their ideas to many research programmes.

## Things to consider when identifying problems that need researching

In general, selecting a researchable problem is about three things:

1. Noticing a gap in the knowledge base, either in the literature or in your clinical knowledge, which cannot be filled by reading or asking others.
2. Having an idea for a research project that could fill that gap.
3. Developing the idea if you are going to undertake the research, often with help from others, into a realistic research question and proposal.

Think about factors that could influence the identification of problems for research. Some of these factors are presented in Box 5.4. Can you add others to this list?

Once you have identified the general area for your research it's important to try to answer the following questions since answering them may help you to judge the extent to which pursuing any area of research is worthwhile.

- Is this problem really important to the delivery of effective nursing, midwifery or health visiting practice?
- Is this problem important to the wider healthcare agenda?

| Box 5.4 | Factors that may influence the generation and pursuance of ideas for research (adapted from le May 2001) |
|---|---|

- A lack of available knowledge about how to deal with a particular problem – this could be either a clinical or an organizational problem.
- Your own experience – perhaps of not knowing the best way to practise or finding that traditional practice does not work.
- Mistakes, complaints or poor practice that lead you to ask whether there is a better way to do things.
- Good practice that could be rolled out to others if there was an evidence base to support it.
- The potential for practice development or enhancement from finding out what works well and how to spread that message.
- Policy – local, national or international – that needs a firmer research base.
- Colleagues and students who help you see the potential of ideas for research.
- Role models who inspire you.
- Service users/patients and carers/relatives who would benefit from better care if your research ideas came to fruition.
- Funding bodies or sponsors who might accept or reject your ideas.
- The last piece of research that you read, heard about or were involved in.
- Undertaking a course which requires you to engage with research.

- To what extent can you research this problem?
- How much support will others give you in terms of resource, time or advice?
- Do you have enough experience to tackle this?
- Do you know of others who might be able to collaborate with you?
- Is the research ethical? (Burns and Grove 2011)

Exercise 5.1 is designed to get you to think about some ideas for research and start to determine whether or not they can feasibly be taken forward as research projects.

### Exercise 5.1  Identifying problems for research

Write a list of problems to which you would like to find solutions or know more about. Once you've completed this, reflect on the potential for turning each of these into a research project. Use the format presented in Figure 5.1 and the questions presented above to help you.

| Problems | Reasons for pursuing your idea | Reasons for abandoning your idea |
| --- | --- | --- |
|  |  |  |

**Figure 5.1** Recording problems for research and determining their feasibility

Now compare your reasons for pursuing or abandoning your idea with some that I have highlighted below:

- personal reasons such as energy levels, motivation, morale and enthusiasm;
- economic reasons related to accessibility and amount of funding;
- resource reasons related to people, time, appropriate technologies, skills and knowledge;
- political reasons which may be local or national;
- ethical reasons related to the nature of the problem and the likely participants in the research. (le May 2001)

To what extent do you agree with these?

Once you have decided that your idea is worth pursuing it is time to consider how to frame the research question(s) that you would like to try to answer. It is also important, at this time, to recognize that you might not end up with a complete, or satisfactory, answer to your question. Some research studies generate only partial answers – which is why there is always potential for more research!

## ■ Getting the question right

Getting the question right requires a particular blend of logical thought, insight, objectivity, practicality and inspiration. In order to do this successfully you might try to use the following step-by-step, reflective approach (based on le May 2001). These steps entail:

1. Deciding on an initial question and ensuring that it reflects the problem or area of concern initially identified. This is critical because the easiest way to waste time and money is by asking the wrong question(s).

2. Searching and appraising the literature (and other sources of evidence including expert knowledge) to see whether the question has already been answered (or is being

researched by someone else). To help you do this, look at the checklists available on the Critical Appraisal Skills Programme (CASP) page of the Solutions for Public Health website: www.sph.nhs.uk/what-we-do/public-health-workforce/resources/. You can find out what research is also being done, or has recently been completed, and is of relevance to health by visiting the National Research Register (NRR) (www.dh.gov.uk/en/Aboutus/Researchanddevelopment/AtoZ/DH_4002357) or the web pages of the NIHR programmes listed in Box 5.2, page 57. If you're interested in research related to social care, visit the Social Care Institute for Excellence's (SCIE) Research Register for Social Care at www.researchregister.org.uk/.

3. Deciding whether the question, once answered, will have clinical relevance. Clinically relevant research questions should:

   a. reflect the reality of practice;
   b. influence the development of practice;
   c. focus on current, or likely future, practice issues;
   d. clearly seek to benefit recipients of care or those involved in its delivery;
   e. be cognisant of the opportunities and constraints to the implementation of any potential findings.

4. Defining each element to be studied within the question to lessen ambiguity and determine whether or not the question can be realistically answered. Each question should address a single issue (Burnard and Morrison 1990), meaning that some projects will have several research questions, since trying to address more than one issue in a question can lead to confusion. A good place to start is to list all the elements that are in your research question to check that they actually reflect the area you wish to study. It is also useful to revisit these elements when you're analysing the data to ensure that you remain focused on finding an answer to your question.

5. Refining and sharpening the question through consultation with peers, experts, service users and any knowledge (published or unpublished) which is already available. It is important to undertake this step in order to reflect on your question's focus and relevance. Systematically accessing and appraising the literature plays an important part in refining questions and checking, again, that no one has answered them already. Drawing together this literature and knowledge in a short summary will be useful in providing a justification for your research and how and where you think your work might fit into the larger picture.

6. Revisiting the question to check whether it really can be researched.

7. Finalizing the question and thinking about how to design a study in order to answer it.

### Exercise 5.2  Turning problems into researchable questions

Take one of the problem areas you identified in Exercise 5.1 and turn it into a researchable question. When you have decided on the initial question, define each element of it and refine and sharpen it through consultation with a variety of sources (peers, experts, consumers, literature, etc.). Note down each of these and consider how they have helped you to become more focused.

Next, consider whether it really is researchable. Use these questions to help you.

- Is there anything to stop you researching this topic after all?
- Is there any likelihood of you finding an answer or increasing your knowledge?
- Do you have the skills and resources to continue?
- Do you have the energy to get started?
- Do you have support for this endeavour?
- Who will benefit from finding an answer to this question?
- Are there any risks associated with finding an answer to this question?

Your end result should be a clearly defined question which we will revisit in subsequent exercises.

Now that you have a better idea about how to devise worthwhile research questions we can move on to consider which research designs and methods for data collection and analysis to use in order to find answers to these questions. The next two chapters will begin to address these important aspects of research.

# ■ References

Burnard P, Morrison P. *Nursing Research in Action*. First edition. 1990; Basingstoke: Macmillan.

Burns N, Grove S. *Understanding Nursing Research: Building an evidence-based practice*. 2011; Maryland Heights, MO: Elsevier Saunders.

le May A. *Making Use of Research*. 2001; London: South Bank University, Distance Learning Centre.

Lloyd K, White J. Democratizing clinical research. *Nature*. 2011; **474**(7351): 277–278.

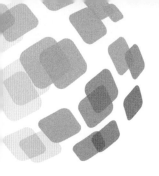

# Chapter 6

# Selecting the right research design to answer your question

## ■ Introduction

In Chapter 5 we thought about writing research questions in order to address clinical problems. Once a question has been set the next stage of the research process is to work out how to answer it. This involves selecting the right research design and methods to generate and analyse the data that will lead you towards an answer. This chapter explores a variety of research designs, while Chapter 7 explores methods which you could use to gather and interpret data and the ideas and rules that underpin them. Knowing these things will help you to select the right research design to answer your question.

## ■ Underpinning perspectives

Research designs, like many elements of life, are structured by a variety of beliefs, values and rules. For some people these are very narrow and focused; for others they take a more eclectic shape, blending a variety of perspectives. These perspectives are often referred to as 'paradigms' and structure not only our understanding of research designs and their applicability but also the meanings and values given to certain types of knowledge, gained through research, within the wider socio-political context of practice.

Paradigms were defined by Kuhn (1962) as a way in which communities of scientists saw the world. They tell us:

- what is important;
- what is legitimate;

- what is reasonable; and
- what to do

within our world (Patton 1978), thereby generating structure and certainty. Paradigms are also associated with power and authority in relation to what is seen as true and what is not. This leads to competition between them and, in turn, influences the sorts of research that we trust to influence our practice (see Chapter 5).

Research designs are situated in a variety of paradigms. In nursing research there are three key paradigms:

- positivism;
- naturalism;
- critical theory.

Each has its own philosophical underpinnings, uniquely linked research designs, and rules that structure specific approaches to the collection and analysis of data. These associated structures guide research and are therefore essential to our understanding of the nature and substance of the research process itself and the findings it generates. However, they do not always act as complementary forces which guide research or practice; more often than not these three paradigms are seen as offering three discrete, often competing rather than informing, views (Kuhn 1962). This incoherence allows supporters to engage in what Oakley (2000) termed 'paradigm wars', in an attempt to secure the superiority of one worldview over another. These debates reflect the variation of their underpinning philosophies. Each, though, has a place to play in guiding research, the development of knowledge and its application to practice and therefore will be considered in more detail below.

> **Exercise 6.1  The three paradigms**
>
> Jot down anything that you know about the three paradigms mentioned above. Refer to your answers as you build up your knowledge of paradigms by reading the next section.

## ■ The three key paradigms

### Positivism

Traditionally positivism is seen as the oldest of these worldviews, with its links to 18th- and 19th-century natural science. Chalmers (1990 p3) suggests that this paradigm emerged in an attempt to 'defend science and to distinguish it from metaphysical and religious discourse', thereby enhancing its credibility. During the 1920s and 1930s, a group of philosophers, known as the Vienna Circle, debated and sharpened this earlier view of science in order to establish a general definition of positivism that could be associated with methods for data collection, analysis and appraisal (Chalmers 1990). Several writers have described the salient features that immediately characterize positivism – you can see these in Box 6.1.

| Box 6.1 | The salient features of positivism |
| --- | --- |

- The ability to make generalizations.
- Objectivity associated with the ability of the researcher to distance him/herself from the focus of the research. This is achieved through the elimination of researcher-focused bias, which is traditionally achieved by the use of standardized research techniques and measurement tools.
- The use of logical reasoning.
- The notion of theory testing rather than theory construction.
- A reliance on the senses, particularly those associated with observation.
- The adoption of a reductionist approach that focuses on the component parts of, for instance, a person rather than taking a more holistic view.

It has become increasingly recognized that these features are associated with an ideal rather than a real set of circumstances and a notable critique has developed suggesting that the basic tenets of positivism may in some instances be deficient or even flawed. A good example of this would be the general use of results from clinical trials which are obtained within highly controlled parameters which often do not mirror the complexities of practice. Box 6.2 gives you a clinical example of this.

| Box 6.2 | Clinical example |
| --- | --- |

Consider the care of an older person with multiple pathology who is taking many different types of medications. The team of healthcare workers looking after this person will rely on the best evidence from clinical trials to support their decisions to prescribe treatments. However, these trials have strict entry criteria and so may not have included people from this age group with co-morbidity; the research evidence is therefore based on a trial that actually excludes patients like this. It may, therefore, fail to give a true picture of the effectiveness and drug interactions which may accompany complex treatment.

One possible solution is to find out whether there are other research studies from other paradigms or research designs that have focused on older people with similar problems, which might provide useful information. Another solution might be to draw on the results of audits of similar people with similar problems.

Despite this disadvantage, clinical trials do give us an indication of what might work, especially if the conditions within which we practise are close enough to those under which the experiment was conducted.

Positivism provides us with one way to view the world and conduct research within it. There has been, however, increased dissatisfaction with this worldview – a feeling that this is not the only way and perhaps not always the best way to answer complex clinical research questions. Positivism can provide only some of the answers needed since it fails to explore the more subjective, less tangible elements of the often messy and complex realities of life at either a collective or an individual level. This recognition of the limitations of positivism spawned an alternative – the naturalistic view.

## Naturalism

The goals of naturalism focus on understanding and interpreting human experience at what may be seen by some as a micro level. This exploration is undertaken without manipulation or control within the natural context of its occurrence. Naturalism is often thought of as being completely opposed to positivism and therefore is seen as competing with the knowledge gained through positivistic enquiry rather than adding to the general body of knowledge that is needed for practice. Many criticize research undertaken within this paradigm as being less structured and so less reliable than that from the positivistic paradigm; however, those critics fail to see that structure is not lessened in this paradigm – merely constructed differently.

Naturalism is frequently described as being holistic and humanistic (De Poy and Gitlin 1994), with the emphasis placed firmly on the exploration of meaning and complexity. You can see the salient features of this worldview in Box 6.3.

---

**Box 6.3    The salient features of naturalism**

- Emphasis is placed on the value of undertaking research in the context within which it is occurring (i.e. the natural setting).
- The ability to describe phenomena in depth.
- Linkage between the world being researched and the researcher's ideas and perceptions of the world; this characteristic often leads to the accusation of subjectivity.
- The notion of interpretation by the researcher and, in some instances, movement towards shared meanings between the researcher and participants in the research (leads to the use of the term 'interpretistic' within this paradigm).
- Generation/construction of new theories or expansion of existing theories rather than testing of theories.
- The adoption of a holistic approach that values the informant as central to the process and acknowledges the context within which their experiences are structured. The emphasis on the social construction of experience (i.e. social, political and economic influences) leads to the association of the term 'constructivism' with this paradigm.

---

## Critical theory

The third paradigm, critical theory, is often thought of as simply a reaction to the constraints of positivism; however, this is an oversimplification. The development of critical theory was influenced by a number of factors, including:

- the oppressive effects of society on the working classes;
- the realization that Marxist views needed modernizing;
- the uncritical nature of the views held by positivists regarding their situation and thereby the perpetuation of the status quo.

The roots of this paradigm stem from a group of scholars working during the 1960s at the Institute of Social Research in Frankfurt University. They began to construct a view of the constraining forces within society which were expressed through:

- *the theory of false consciousness* in which the self-understandings of a group of people may be false or lack coherence;
- *the theory of crisis* in which crisis threatens the social cohesiveness of a group of people and therefore becomes a threat to the group's integrity;
- *the theory of education* in which the emphasis is placed on the benefits of knowledge;
- *the theory of transformative action* which details the need for actions to ensure that change is made and acted upon (Manias and Street 2000 p51).

This movement led to the development of a number of critical theories that include feminist approaches and participatory action research and are characterized by:

- recognition of the importance of the social, economic and political processes of society;
- their focus on enlightenment, empowerment and emancipation;
- the aim of transforming existing social order by focusing on power relationships and using self-reflection;
- the provision of explanations through exploration of the effects of knowledge, power and values.

Although relatively young, this paradigm is increasingly finding favour within the nursing professions for the following reasons:

- the focus on practice and potential to be transformational;
- the fit between its emancipatory and empowering nature and the notion of nursing being an emergent profession which was (and may continue to be) dominated by the more positivistic model espoused by medicine;
- the clear articulation of equality between the researcher and those being researched. This approach complements health and social care policies that focus increasingly on developing and sustaining patient and professional partnerships.

### Exercise 6.2  Fitting within a paradigm

Think of an issue related to your practice and find a research paper addressing this topic. Read the paper and decide which paradigm it fits within. Then decide whether the topic could fall within the boundaries of either of the other worldviews. If it would, how would you alter the research question to fit with the salient features of the other paradigms?

## *Towards a paradigm merger – mixed methods*

Given the complex nature of life and people it is not surprising that there is a movement towards an alternative, more eclectic, approach to research which merges the best of the paradigms rather than seeing them as competing with, or excluding, each other. This mixing may benefit both the development of knowledge and its application to practice. The best known of these more eclectic approaches is known simply as mixed methods (Creswell and Plano Clark 2007). Mixed methods studies usually combine research designs and their associated methods from the positivistic and naturalistic paradigms in one study in order to use the findings from one to complement or explain the other. The purpose of this combination is to answer comprehensively some of the questions raised in practice.

## *Other paradigms – qualitative and quantitative: a cautionary note*

Although the three paradigms highlighted above are the driving forces behind research, you commonly hear about two more worldviews: the qualitative and the quantitative paradigms. These terms have attracted much attention in recent years, leading to their growth from simple descriptors of data generated within particular paradigms (i.e. qualitative data – presented largely as words – and quantitative data – presented largely as numbers) into paradigms in their own right. Establishing these two data types as discrete paradigms is a little confusing since neither is associated with a set of theoretical or methodological assumptions (Atkinson 1995) such as those we have already seen with positivism, naturalism and critical theory.

## ■ How things fit together – paradigms, designs, methods and data

The next thing we need to consider is how the three main paradigms fit with study designs, the methods used to collect information (data) and the types of data that are produced. These relationships are highlighted in Table 6.1 (the methods mentioned in the table are discussed in detail in Chapter 7).

At first this may appear confusing since you probably think that some worldviews will exclude certain methods for collecting data; however, as you can see from Table 6.1, this is not the case. For instance, observation and interviewing can be used across all paradigms and designs: their versatility is associated with the amount of structure researchers impose on them – less structure makes them useful in the naturalistic and critical theory paradigms (e.g. unstructured or semi-structured interviews); more structure makes them useful for collecting data to be quantified in experimental and survey designs (e.g. structured interviews or observations that are based around a pre-determined schedule).

**Table 6.1** How things fit together

| Paradigm | Design examples | Methods of data collection | Types of data generated |
|---|---|---|---|
| Positivism | Experiments (true and quasi)<br>Surveys | Observation<br>Measurement scales<br>Questionnaires | Mainly quantitative |
| Naturalism | Ethnography<br>Phenomenology<br>Case studies | Observation<br>Interviews | Mainly qualitative |
| Critical theory | Action research | Observation<br>Interviews | Both quantitative and qualitative |

# ■ Research designs

An understanding of the variety of research designs and methods for collecting and analysing data is essential to both the generation and use of research findings. This section outlines the major designs that you will come into contact with; the details of the principal methods of data collection used in these designs in healthcare are discussed in Chapter 7 together with an overview of the ways in which data collected through these methods can be analysed and understood. You will also find in this section criteria to help you judge the worth of research presented within the major designs and therefore its applicability to practice.

> **Exercise 6.3  Choosing research designs**
>
> As you read this section, revisit the research question you generated in Chapter 5 and consider how you could design a study using each of the research designs discussed below to help you to answer that question. Reflect on the ability of each design to provide you with different types of information (qualitative and quantitative) and decide which would be the best design to choose.

The most popular research designs are:

- experiments (true and quasi);
- surveys;
- ethnography;
- phenomenology;
- case study;
- action research.

As we have already seen, each design is linked to an explicit worldview, associated with specific methods for data collection and generating certain types of data more readily than others (see Table 6.1). In this section we will consider what each of the designs listed above is, what their most important characteristics are and how you can judge their worth.

## *The experiment*

There are two design alternatives within this tradition:

- the true experiment;
- the quasi-experiment.

Their differences relate simply to the presence or absence of one or more of a set of attributes. Therefore, for an experiment to be classified as true, it must incorporate each of the following attributes:

1. manipulation;
2. control;
3. randomization.

If any are missing it becomes quasi – not quite true.

In order to understand the inherent principles of the experimental design, each of these attributes needs elaboration.

Manipulation of an independent variable is a key component within the true experimental design and refers to the testing of the effectiveness of an intervention through its administration to one group (usually known as the experimental group) and comparison with the outcomes of a group which has not been subjected to the intervention (the control group). In other words, the independent variable is manipulated either by having it absent or present (De Poy and Gitlin 1994); its effectiveness is determined through the comparison of the groups when the dependent variable (i.e. the effect) is assessed.

Control simply means the existence of a group in which the independent variable is withheld (the control group); this usually means that this group, when we are referring to research in health and social care, receives the usual care and so is not disadvantaged in any way. This facet of the experimental design enables researchers to determine the effectiveness of an intervention since control and experimental groups are usually matched as closely as possible to allow the meaningful comparison of findings to be made between the two.

Randomization is the allocation of participants to one or other group within the experiment (i.e. the control or experimental group). This can occur either at the sample selection phase or the group allocation stage (De Poy and Gitlin 1994). The more sophisticated approach is to randomly allocate at the sample selection phase, which minimizes bias, ensures that every participant has an equal chance of being in either group and therefore adds strength to the notion of generalizability.

True experiments contain all the above attributes – manipulation, control and randomization. Quasi-experiments, meanwhile, have one attribute missing, usually because it is deemed to be unethical or unrealistic to withhold an intervention or use randomization.

Both types of experiment are frequently used in health and social care research. Their advantages and disadvantages are presented in Table 6.2. Despite some disadvantages, many researchers choose this approach above all others. The relevance of findings generated using experimental designs should not be underestimated.

**Table 6.2** Advantages and disadvantages of experimental type designs

| Advantages | Disadvantages |
|---|---|
| • The ability to determine causality – the effect of one thing on another.<br><br>• The ability to generalize from the research sample to the larger population.<br><br>• Repeatability given the same set of circumstances.<br><br>• Precision and minimization of bias. | • Ethically it may be inappropriate to withhold interventions or knowledge about which group people belong to (this is particularly important in drug trials when placebo medication is given).<br><br>• Transferring the findings from the artificially constructed experiment into the realities of practice may be impractical.<br><br>• Recruiting enough people to form control and experimental groups of sufficient size to achieve meaningful results can be problematic.<br><br>• Control of variables may not always be possible. |

**Exercise 6.4  Experiments: thinking about evaluation**

Think about how you would evaluate research generated through the experimental type designs. Write down six of your own criteria against which to evaluate this type of research, then compare them with the criteria below and the Critical Appraisal Skills Programme (CASP) appraisal tool for randomized controlled trials (RCTs), which can be found at **www.sph.nhs. uk/sph-files/casp-appraisal-tools/S.Reviews%20Appraisal%20Tool.pdf/view.**

## Criteria against which experimental designs may be evaluated

Crombie (1996) identified several criteria that will allow us to make an assessment, or appraisal, of the value of data generated through the true experimental design. These include the following questions:

- Was there random allocation to interventions?
- How was the randomization carried out?
- Were the groups comparable at the start?

- Could the selection of participants influence the size of the effect of the treatment?
- Were all the participants accounted for?
- Were those who withdrew from the study different to those remaining in the study to the end?
- Were there any ambiguities in the description of the intervention and/or its administration?
- Were the outcomes of the interventions assessed without the researcher knowing which group was receiving the intervention (blind assessment)?
- Could bias have been introduced, e.g. through lack of blind assessment?
- Were any deviations from the intervention protocol reported?
- Were any side effects reported?

## The survey

The survey is sometimes referred to as a non-experimental design since it relies on statistical manipulation of data rather than the actual manipulation of interventions so important to the experimental design. The survey does fall within the same paradigm as the experiment, however, and is therefore directed by the same principles (see Box 6.1, page 65). Surveys are useful and flexible designs, typically conducted on large numbers of people, to describe the characteristics of a population and/or predict its behaviour(s) through the generation of both quantitative and qualitative data.

There are several types of survey commonly used across the health and social care arena. The main ones are:

- descriptive surveys, which provide a complete description of the population or phenomenon under study;
- comparative surveys, which compare information gained from one group with another;
- longitudinal surveys, which are undertaken over long periods of time and allow researchers to detail change or trends over time;
- correlational surveys, which describe relationships and determine whether there are any positive or negative correlations between them.

Although a well-used design, there are associated advantages and disadvantages that need to be considered (see Table 6.3).

### Exercise 6.5  Surveys: thinking about evaluation

Think about how you would evaluate research generated through surveys. Write down six of your own criteria against which to evaluate this type of design, then compare with the criteria below.

**Table 6.3** Advantages and disadvantages of surveys

| Advantages | Disadvantages |
|---|---|
| • The ability to collect data from large numbers of people.<br><br>• The ability to generalize from the research sample to the larger population.<br><br>• Repeatability given the same set of circumstances.<br><br>• Cost-effectiveness.<br><br>• The provision of anonymity to participants.<br><br>• A variety of variables can be targeted within the survey and the dataset produced can be analysed in many different ways. | • The possibility of non-response.<br><br>• The complexity of the data-collecting instruments and the need to be unambiguous if questionnaires are used.<br><br>• Interviews with large numbers of people may be expensive and minimize the feeling of anonymity transferred through the questionnaire.<br><br>• Respondents, if anonymous, cannot be followed up.<br><br>• Responses may not be accurate. |

### Criteria against which survey designs may be evaluated

Crombie (1996) highlights several questions that we can use to assess the trustworthiness of findings generated by surveys. He carefully points out that their versatility can also lead to their abuse and therefore their results need careful appraisal.

- Who was studied?
- How was the sample obtained?
- What was the response rate?
- Was the design appropriate to meet the purpose of the survey?
- How well planned was the survey?
- Were the findings serendipitous?
- Can the results be generalized?
- Did anything unusual occur within the study?
- Do all the numbers add up and how are data presented?
- How are the findings interpreted in relation to the initial aims of the survey?

## Ethnography

Fetterman (1998 p1) describes ethnography as 'the art and science of describing a group or culture' regardless of location – a far-off land or a hospital ward. The salient features of ethnography are:

- the construction of a rich description of the culture or group which is focused on a selected problem or topic of interest;
- the use of observation, records and interviews to develop this picture;

- the ability of the researcher to determine the credibility of one person's opinions against others;
- the ability to collect data 'in the field' and continue to analyse it once one has left the culture or group under study;
- the ability to keep an open mind and write up the story without distortion or manipulation.

The advantages and disadvantages of this research design are presented in Table 6.4.

**Table 6.4**  Advantages and disadvantages of ethnography

| Advantages | Disadvantages |
|---|---|
| • The ability to observe situations as they occur. | • The researcher's view of reality becomes distorted because they become so engrossed in the situation they are studying. |
| • The provision of rich, detailed descriptions which allow the realities and subtleties of the culture to be exposed. | • The potential to fail to capture the entire picture, presenting rather a series of disjointed sections. |
| • The completeness of the description. | |
| • The ability of the account to be seen as a description of that particular group but also the possibility of others seeing similarities with their own cultures within it. | • Failure to move from the description to the analytic. |
| | • Ethical questions may be raised with respect to the intrusion on privacy necessitated by the ethnographer. |
| • The ability of this approach to harness the uniqueness of individual perspectives and how people act within their worlds. | • Access may be difficult since many people will not want to expose themselves to the depth of enquiry necessitated by this design. |
| • The explicit nature of the researcher within this design and the inherent value of this. | • An inability of the ethnographer to see the obvious – making the mundane new is central to complete description. |
| • The presence of the researcher should impact minimally on the setting, thereby retaining the notion of naturalness. | |

### Exercise 6.6  Ethnography: thinking about evaluation

Think about how you would evaluate research generated through ethnography. Write down six of your own criteria against which to evaluate this type of research, then compare them with the criteria below.

## Criteria against which ethnographies may be evaluated

Denscombe (1998) provides a useful checklist for ethnographic research that could be used to determine the value of research findings from ethnographies:

- Has the naturalness of the setting been maintained?
- Has the research been conducted ethically?
- Has access to the setting been gained appropriately?
- Has a holistic approach been adopted linking data coherently?

- Has sufficient time been allowed to collect enough information to provide a rich description of the group or culture?
- Does the researcher provide a description of his/her role in the research?
- Does the researcher acknowledge the level of interpretation involved in the process of description?
- Are the findings compared and contrasted with findings from other similar ethnographies?

## Phenomenology

Moustakas (1994 p84) suggests that 'evidence from phenomenological research is derived from first-person reports of life experiences'. This evidence helps us to understand the experiences of others and the meanings that they attribute to them – in other words, 'it is a way of seeing the world through another person's eyes' (Stephenson and Corben 1997 p115) and is therefore very useful in helping us to illuminate practice-related issues.

Phenomenological approaches stem from the work of two German philosophers – Husserl (1859–1938) and his pupil Heidegger (1889–1976). Each took a slightly different approach. Husserl preferred to describe phenomena with minimal interpretation, believing that the purity of the description was dependent on the researcher being able to set aside (or bracket) their pre-suppositions in relation to the area of investigation, thereby articulating only the experiences of the participants. Heidegger, meanwhile, moved away from this, taking a more interpretive stance which acknowledges the researcher's background and inherent knowledge of the phenomenon; in doing this there is an interpretation of the participant's experience which is in some way framed by the researcher's exposure to his/her own world. Thus these two approaches have become known as:

- descriptive phenomenology (Husserlian)
- interpretative phenomenology (Heideggerian).

Despite their differences they share some of the salient features implicit in the exploration and articulation of others' experiences, placing the emphasis firmly on 'the nature of being, the here and now, "as it is"' (Stephenson and Corben 1997 p117).

Phenomenological research is typified by:

- its emphasis on experience as it is *now*;
- its concern to understand the phenomenon as it is without manipulation through the consideration of:
  - the way people exist in the world;
  - the significance of everyday things and events;
  - the essential ingredients of the phenomenon.

However, as with all designs, phenomenology has its associated advantages and disadvantages (see Table 6.5).

**Table 6.5**  Advantages and disadvantages of phenomenology

| Advantages | Disadvantages |
|---|---|
| • Enhances our understanding of everyday experiences. | • The risk of misrepresenting the phenomenon. |
| • Provides an approach which facilitates the systematic collection of information about how people experience phenomena. | • The risk of presenting incomplete findings. |
| | • The inability to generalize from the experiences explored. |
| • The completeness of the description of the phenomenon. | • The risk of exploring experiences which make participants vulnerable. |
| • The ability for others to recognize their experience from the accounts of the participants – transferability or resonance. | |

### Exercise 6.7  Phenomenology: thinking about evaluation

Think about how you would evaluate research generated through phenomenological designs. Write down six of your own criteria against which to evaluate this type of research, then compare them with the criteria below.

## Criteria against which phenomenology may be evaluated

This design has great potential within the nursing professions. However, it is essential that we are able to assess the quality of the findings generated through this approach. The following requirements of phenomenological research have been proposed by Annells (1999) in order to help us to do this:

- an understandable account of the phenomenon;
- an understandable process of enquiry – a clear decision trail;
- a useful product which has the potential to inform practice;
- an appropriate approach to the enquiry – descriptive or interpretative;
- a sound linkage between methods for data collection and analysis and the findings.

## *Case studies*

Case studies are used widely in health and social care research. This approach tends to cluster together several techniques applied within other research designs (e.g. interviews, observations, surveys, documentary analysis). Their uniqueness is in this clustering. Denscombe (1998) describes the salient characteristics of case studies as:

- the focus on just one instance of the thing that is to be investigated – the case;
- the notion of an in-depth study of that case – the focus is on the particular rather than the general;

- the possibility of gaining unique and valuable insights related to that case;
- the focus on relationships and processes within the case which tend to be interconnected and interrelated rather than solely based on outcomes;
- the possibility of completeness;
- the naturalness of the research – manipulation is absent;
- the use of multiple sources of data and multiple methods to tap these.

The greatest challenge for researchers using this design is the selection of the case – to what extent will it be typical or extreme? How representative will the case be? What are the boundaries to the case? Each of these questions must be considered before this design is utilized. There are, however, other disadvantages and indeed advantages to this design, detailed in Table 6.6.

**Table 6.6**  Advantages and disadvantages of case study design

| Advantages | Disadvantages |
|---|---|
| • The potential for in-depth information to be generated which captures the subtleties and intricacies of each case.<br><br>• The possibility of using several methods for the collection (and analysis) of data to either present the entire picture or confirm results gained from one method with those gained from another.<br><br>• The potential for using this design to test or generate theory. | • The risks associated with generalization.<br><br>• Maintaining the boundaries of the case.<br><br>• Negotiating access to the multiple sources of data that are needed to present a full picture of the case.<br><br>• The influence of the researcher on the case. |

**Exercise 6.8  Case studies: thinking about evaluation**

Think about how you would evaluate research generated through case study designs. Write down six of your own criteria against which to evaluate this type of research, then compare them with the criteria below.

## Criteria against which case studies may be evaluated

Denscombe (1998) also offers us a set of questions against which to judge case study research, which include:

- Have the criteria for selection of the case(s) been made explicit?
- Is the case a self-contained entity?
- Is the case identifiable?
- Is the research naturalistic?
- Have the boundaries of the case been described?
- Have the significant features of the case been described and where appropriate compared with similar cases?

- Does the research make use of multiple methods for data collection and multiple sources of data?
- Does the research present the entire picture?

## *Action research*

This design has been attracting more and more interest within the nursing profession in recent years and yet it is hard to find a clear definition of what it actually entails. Without the clarity of one single definition it is best to conceptualize action research as a design that must be:

- practical (action focused – dealing with real-world situations);
- change oriented;
- cyclical, ensuring feedback between cycles which drives future change. Each cycle comprises elements of reflection, evaluation and subsequent use of findings to progress future actions;
- participatory – participation is active rather than passive and emphasizes the equality of the relationship between the researcher and the participant.

Set against this background there are several challenges that the action research team needs to be aware of. These include the ownership of the research and the ethics associated with the process of action research. These ethical problems focus on (Winter 1996 p17):

- driving forces within the study – there is a need for the development of the work to remain visible and open to suggestions from others. Failure to do this may redistribute power balances and minimize the potential for equality and empowerment linked to this design;
- permission to access multiple sources of data;
- description of others' work and views – this may pose problems related to confidentiality and anonymity throughout the project and at publication.

Selection of this design needs careful consideration – it is not one for novices and despite its seductive nature there remain several disadvantages as well as advantages (see Table 6.7).

> **Exercise 6.9  Action research: thinking about evaluation**
>
> Think about how you would evaluate research generated through action research. Write down six of your own criteria against which to evaluate this type of research, then compare them with the criteria below.

**Table 6.7** Advantages and disadvantages of action research

| Advantages | Disadvantages |
|---|---|
| • The potential to address practical issues.<br><br>• The cyclical and participatory nature of this design means that research findings can be rapidly incorporated into practice.<br><br>• It involves practitioners not only in the process of change but also in the design and execution of research. | • The findings from this design are likely to be unique to those participating – generalization is not possible.<br><br>• The ownership of the research is ambiguous.<br><br>• The motives of the researcher may limit the potential of empowerment and emancipation associated with this design.<br><br>• Undertaking action research presents an 'extra' burden to practitioners above and beyond their normal work patterns.<br><br>• The researcher is unlikely to be able to remain detached and objective. |

### Criteria against which action research may be evaluated
- Does the research address a particular issue?
- Is there participation at all stages of the project?
- Have ground rules been set for participation?
- Is the research part of a process for development or a one-off instance?
- Is there a strategy for maintaining change when the research finishes?
- Is there a mechanism for feeding findings back to participants on an ongoing basis?
- Have ethical considerations been taken into account?
- Is the research able to be combined with the realities of practice? (Denscombe 1998 p67)

Now that you are more familiar with the three key research paradigms and the designs associated with them we will move on, in the next chapter, to think more precisely about how you can collect and analyse data.

## ■ Further reading

Appleton J. Critiquing approaches to case study design for a constructivist inquiry. *Qualitative Research Journal.* 2002; **2**(2): 80–97.

Meyer J. Action research. In: K Gerrish, A Lacey (eds). *The Research Process in Nursing.* 2010; Oxford: Wiley-Blackwell.

Smith G. Experiments. In: R Watson, H McKenna, S Cowman, J Keady (eds). *Nursing Research: Designs and methods.* 2008; Edinburgh: Churchill Livingstone.

# ■ References

Annells M. Evaluating phenomenology: usefulness, quality and philosophical foundations. *Nurse Researcher.* 1999; **6**(3): 5–19.

Atkinson P. Pearls, pith and provocation: some perils of paradigms. *Qualitative Health Research.* 1995; **5**(1): 117–124.

Chalmers A. *Science and its Fabrication.* 1990; Milton Keynes: Open University Press.

Creswell J, Plano Clark V. *Designing and Conducting Mixed Methods Research.* 2007; Thousand Oaks, CA: Sage.

Crombie I. *The Pocket Guide to Critical Appraisal.* 1996; London: BMJ Publishing Group.

De Poy E, Gitlin L. *Introduction to Research. Understanding and applying multiple strategies.* 1994; St Louis, MO: Mosby.

Denscombe M. *The Good Research Guide for Small Scale Social Research Projects.* 1998; Buckingham: Open University Press.

Fetterman D. *Ethnography.* 1998; Thousand Oaks, CA: Sage Publications.

Kuhn T. *The Structure of Scientific Revolutions.* 1962; Chicago: University of Chicago Press.

Manias E, Street A. Possibilities for critical social theory and Foucault's work: a toolbox approach. *Nursing Inquiry.* 2000; **7**(1): 50–60.

Moustakas C. *Phenomenological Research Methods.* 1994; Thousand Oaks, CA: Sage.

Oakley A. *Experiments in Knowing.* 2000; Cambridge: Polity Press.

Patton M. *Utilization-Focused Evaluation.* 1978; Beverly Hills, CA: Sage Publications.

Stephenson N, Corben V. Phenomenology. In: P Smith (ed.). *Research Mindedness for Practice.* 1997; Edinburgh: Churchill Livingstone.

Winter R. Some principles and procedures for the conduct of action research. In: O Zuber-Skerritt (ed.). *New Directions in Action Research.* 1996; London: Falmer Press.

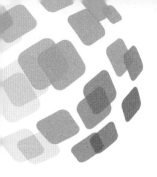

# Chapter 7

# Collecting and analysing data – some important principles

## ■ Introduction

In Chapter 6 you read about research paradigms and designs. This chapter focuses on particular methods for collecting and analysing data. First, it explores the most common methods of data collection that can be used in the research designs explored in Chapter 6. Second, it focuses on some of the fundamental principles underlying the analysis of quantitative and qualitative data. It concludes with a section considering how you can judge whether the research that you read about can be trusted enough to implement in practice.

## ■ Methods for collecting data

We will start with experimental designs before moving on to focus on interviews, questionnaires and observation.

> **Exercise 7.1  Moving from design to method**
>
> Before reading on, go back to your research question. Think about the designs that you have just read about. Which one would be the most useful to you and which would be the best method for you to use for collecting data?

Here we will consider the principles underpinning each of these methods.

### Experiments and quasi-experiments

In healthcare research these approaches to data collection make carefully structured observations and collect data according to explicit and pre-determined criteria and, as shown in Chapter 6, offer an effective way of establishing causality (cause and effect) due to a high level of control. They can be structured in a number of ways to allow the collection of appropriate and relevant data such as pre-test–post-test designs, cross-over studies or using the patient as their own control.

As we have seen, a true experiment involves random allocation of a representative sample of participants to the experimental or control group; pre-test measurements (observations) are made before the experiment starts to enable the researcher to gain baseline data against which changes can be judged. The intervention is then carried out in the experimental group while the control group receives the usual treatment and gets no experimental intervention. In a cross-over study, patients are allocated to one group and then to the other (crossed over), after a defined period, allowing the findings to be compared, while, when using the patient as their own control, their baseline data is compared with that obtained following the intervention.

In either case, the effectiveness of the intervention is determined by comparing the outcome between the two groups providing quantitative data, which are analysed using inferential statistics (see page 86). The extent of the difference (if any) between the groups on completion of the study indicates the confidence that can be placed in the findings.

In a quasi-experimental design, although an experimental treatment/intervention is introduced, some element of the true experiment is missing. Control may not be possible due to, for example, the nature of the intervention or the characteristics of the participants. In most cases, however, the missing factor is that of randomization. A quasi-experimental design is used in a similar way to the true experiment, though it is associated with weakened confidence in making causal assertions and with a greater level of threat to internal validity.

## Interviews, questionnaires and observational techniques

It is important to remember that any of the three remaining data-collection methods can be used in the six designs we reviewed in Chapter 6. This is because of their inherent flexibility: researchers designing interviews, questionnaires or observations can build into them different amounts of structure, depending on the underlying principles of their study design and their research question. This is why you will hear and read about structured and unstructured interviews or observation and open and closed questions within the framework of a questionnaire. These will be discussed below.

## Interviews

Interviews are a valuable method of collecting information about a variety of topics. They are widely used and offer the potential for a structured approach or for a more fluid, unstructured approach to be adopted. However, they are complex to administer successfully since they involve a variety of skilled behaviours as well as knowledge of the area being researched. The component parts of the interview, regardless of its structure, involve:

- asking questions;
- active listening;
- reflecting on answers and non-verbal cues;
- the skilled use of non-verbal and verbal communication;
- the ability to interpret responses in order to appropriately frame the next question.

Interviewing is a highly skilled endeavour that needs sophisticated planning together with an understanding of how the interviewer can affect both the process and the outcomes. Its versatility is heightened by the potential to undertake interviews at both the individual level, either in person (face to face) or remotely (e.g. over the phone, through video links or electronically), and the group level (e.g. through focus groups).

Denscombe (1998) suggests that interviews can be used in situations when:

- detailed information is required;
- data may be based on sensitive issues, emotions and experiences;
- depth rather than breadth is important in order to answer the research question(s).

### Advantages of interviews
- Potential for the generation of in-depth information.
- Development of insights into others' experiences, emotions and feelings.
- Simplicity in terms of resources.
- Flexibility to reflect on answers and respond accordingly or to rephrase questions to ensure clarity.
- High levels of response.
- Credibility of the data since checking meaning and interpretation is possible.
- Potential for the participants to feel valued and that their views are important.

### Disadvantages of interviews
- Resource intensive in terms of time and researcher energy.
- Large amounts of data will be generated and need to be analysed.
- The interviewer may impact on the process and outcome of the interview, leading to the collection of unreliable data.
- Technical problems associated with audio or video tape recording.
- The potential to unsettle respondents through the personal nature of the interviews or the need to probe beyond the superficial.

## Questionnaires

Questionnaires are perhaps the most used (and abused) method for collecting information. Their attraction centres on their potential to gather written data from large numbers of people in what appears to be a relatively simple way. Their downfall is that the seemingly simple (in terms of question construction and data production) is actually extremely difficult.

Questionnaires are useful in situations that:

- gather data from large numbers of people in a variety of locations;
- require the capture of structured, straightforward information;
- require an element of standardized information (Denscombe 1998).

### Advantages of questionnaires
- Economical.
- Generate large amounts of data across wide sections of the population.
- Allow comparison between groups of people in a standardized way.
- Potential to minimize the effect of the researcher on the data presented.

### Disadvantages of questionnaires
- Risk of poor response rates.
- Risk of incomplete or false answers.
- Can be expensive if distributed and/or returned by post.
- Limited by the researcher's ability to construct relevant unambiguous questions.
- Expensive in terms of researcher time in early stages of questionnaire construction.

## Observation

Observation is about creating a picture of the world that represents reality. It involves watching, listening and interpreting the specific and mundane elements of that world in order to represent them fairly in a final, detailed description. Observers traditionally either participate in the activities being observed (participant observation) or remain on the periphery of the world that they are observing (non-participant). Observation is highly reliant on the researcher, rather than the study participants, to find and report on data since it does not involve the verbal (or written) interactions associated with interviews or questionnaires.

### Advantages of observation
- Potential to gather large amounts of data.
- Independent of participants answering questions.
- Relatively inexpensive in terms of resources.
- Can be used with audio and video recording equipment.
- Allows recording of complete situations.
- Ability to provide in-depth descriptions.

### Disadvantages of observation
- Hard to control for unexpected events.
- Cannot predict occurrence, time or duration of events targeted for observation.

- Bias of personal interpretation.
- Rapid speed of events.
- Some situations are not recordable.
- Anonymity may be hard to ensure.
- Potential for variability between observers.
- Personal involvement of the observer.

## Flexibility within data-collection techniques

We have suggested that each of the principal methods of data collection has potential for use with each research design. This seemingly bizarre statement results from each method's flexibility in terms of structure. Thus the structured interview is useful in the experiment and survey to collect information that can be quantified; the unstructured interview is useful in the collection of free-flowing qualitative information in an ethnographic or phenomenological design. The questionnaire has the same structural properties, while observation, when undertaken as a non-participant, can take on a more structured format and recording mechanism than participant observation.

## Analysing data

There are two overarching types of data generated from research:

- quantitative (primarily numbers)
- qualitative (primarily words).

Both have equal value in enhancing our understanding of the world of health and social care and should be treated as such. Our main challenge, if we want to base practice on sound research, is to understand how to make sense of the information presented to us, either in its raw state (fresh from the data-collection process) or in its analysed state in papers or through other forms of presentation. As students you will be spending most of your time trying to make sense of already analysed data that you have read in papers or research reports.

As you read more widely, you will notice that there are many more approaches used by researchers to analyse quantitative or qualitative data than there are methods to collect these data. This strange phenomenon means that you will often have to look up the details of each specific method used to analyse data in order to fully understand how to use it or how researchers have used it in the papers and research reports that you're reading – it is impossible to hold all this complicated information in your head. Despite this, we think that there are a number of key facts that you need to know.

## Quantitative data

This type of data is numerical and therefore easily analysed using statistics. It is primarily used to examine relationships between and among variables and is central to answering questions and addressing hypotheses obtained through surveys, experiments and quasi-experiments. It is particularly useful for testing cause-and-effect relationships and helps to eliminate alternative explanations. To explain causality requires that three criteria are met:

- there must be a relationship (association) between the causal variable and the effect variable;
- the cause must precede the effect;
- the relationship cannot be explained by another variable.

Two main statistical approaches can be used:

- descriptive statistics;
- inferential statistics.

Descriptive statistics are about describing the features of the data – for example, the overall size of the sample, the characteristics of that group (e.g. the percentage of men and women), the frequency with which something occurred or how certain features are distributed throughout the data set. Often descriptive statistics are presented as text, pie diagrams, graphs and/or bar charts.

Inferential statistics are concerned with making predictions about whether or not certain factors that are found in a small group of participants (a sample) will be found in a larger group (a population) or establishing the relationship between variables. There are specific sets of rules associated with selecting different inferential techniques linked to the size of the sample and the level of the data acquired.

Telling you about the myriad statistical tests available to you and helping you to decide which one to use in which set of circumstances is beyond the scope of this book. Selecting statistical tests is not something that you can do without further help and we advise you to seek out a sympathetic statistician for guidance and find an easy-to-read statistics book (see Further reading, page 90).

## Qualitative data

Qualitative data are words, either spoken or written. Although numerous explicit techniques are used – and associated with the various research designs outlined in Chapter 6 – there is a common general pattern of moving from an individual's description, for example taken from a transcript of an interview, to the researcher's synthesis (bringing together) of all participants' descriptions. This is generally achieved using one of two fundamental ways of making sense of the information obtained:

- classification (Dey 1993); or
- immersion/crystallization (Crabtree and Miller 1992).

Classification (coding) is a way of sorting data systematically into categories. Classification systems may be pre-determined from the literature or may 'emerge' from the data. Once a system has been identified, data are simply slotted into it. Immersion/ crystallization is more nebulous. This process involves a prolonged engagement (immersion) with the text, resulting, after substantial thought and consideration, in a crystallization (coming together) of the ideas held in the text and the formulation of an account describing them. This necessitates careful and repeated reading of the transcripts obtained to identify significant words or phrases and, when all transcripts have been analysed, distilling (crystallizing) them in a way that captures their central (essential) meaning.

When you are undertaking any sort of qualitative data analysis you need to:

- keep focused on your research question(s);
- reflect on the data and discuss it with other people to try to rule out biases and formulate your ideas;
- aim for rich, thick, detailed accounts of the findings, including appropriate quotations from, for example, participant or observational field notes;
- check back with participants, if possible, to ensure that the final account reflects their experiences/views.

These ideas can also be used to guide your critique of qualitative data analysis in papers.

Both quantitative and qualitative data analysis can be done manually or by using a computer program. There are numerous programs available to researchers, but whichever one is used, it will be only as good as the data entered into it – very careful data entry is required to ensure that the results generated are as reliable as they can be.

## ■ Trusting findings: checking reliability, validity and credibility

One of the most important questions that people ask about research is: 'To what extent can I trust these findings?' Certain conventions, linked to the paradigms outlined in Chapter 6, are associated with answering this question, and involve the inclusion of several checks and balances which help researchers to generate trustworthy findings. The terms 'reliability' and 'validity' are conventionally linked to the positivistic paradigm, whereas 'credibility' is routinely associated with the naturalistic and critical theory paradigms.

*Reliability* is the extent to which an experiment, test or other measuring procedure yields the same result when repeated over time, within the same framework of research (Bannigan and Watson 2009). There are various ways to establish this:

1.  Test–retest: this is simply when a test is administered then repeated after a lapse of time to the same sample. The results are then compared to assess the extent of their agreement.

2.  Equivalence testing: this is when two similar tests are administered at the same time and the results compared for agreement, or administration of two forms of the scale to the same sample, successively (alternate form reliability).

3.  Split-half testing: this involves using one test in which each component measures the feature being assessed. When the data are analysed, the results for half of the questions are compared with those from the remaining half. The extent of the agreement is then measured.

In each of these examples a close match in terms of agreement signifies reliability of the data and hence suggests a sound level of trustworthiness.

*Validity* is often thought of as being harder to establish than reliability, although the two are interlinked and one should not be considered without regard to the other. Validity means the extent to which the methods for data collection actually collect data about the issues being investigated – it refers to honesty and accuracy (Lowe 1993). Various types of validity have been discussed in research texts, with the most commonly referred to by researchers being:

- face validity (the extent to which the data-collection methods appear, on the face of it, to be asking the right questions or taking the right measurements);
- content validity (this involves asking experts to verify the questions or measurements that are to be used – judging the relevance of the content of the tests);
- construct validity (this is linked to the components of any underlying theories which have informed the construction of the data-collection tools);
- predictive validity (the extent to which the instruments accurately predict future trends – this involves gathering data at one point in time, then once again to compare predictions with reality);
- concurrent validity (the extent to which findings from two similar tests, if administered concurrently, generate the same results).

A variety of approaches should be used (McDowell and Newell 1996).

You will also find reference to internal and external validity in which internal validity refers to the ability of the research design to accurately answer the research question(s) and external validity refers to the capacity to generalize from the study findings to the larger population (De Poy and Gitlin 1998).

*Credibility* is linked closely with establishing the trustworthiness and accurate representation of views when qualitative data are presented for analysis. De Poy and Gitlin (1998 p305) define credibility as 'truth value and accuracy of findings in naturalistic inquiry'. This process is vital to our understanding of the extent to which the researcher has documented the processes of data collection and analysis as well as the extent to which their interpretation of the data checks out with that of the participants. Techniques for enhancing credibility include:

- triangulation (checking data from one source against data generated through another);
- saturation (refers to the point when the researcher is confident that sufficient data has been generated to answer the research questions);
- member checks (involves asking participants in the study to check their agreement with the researcher's interpretations of the findings);
- reflexivity (is about the researcher being aware and exposing his/her personal biases and assumptions related to the process of the research);
- audit trails (refers to a trail of thinking and rationale for judgements taken as the study progresses);
- peer debriefing (the process of involving peers in the analysis of data – this may involve independent assessment of data and then making a comparison linked to the agreement between assessors) (De Poy and Gitlin 1998).

Alongside these checks, an assessment needs to be made in relation to the clinical relevance of any research findings. The questions in Box 7.1 will help you to make this judgement.

| Box 7.1 | Judging the clinical relevance of research findings (adapted from le May and Gabbay 2011) |
|---|---|

Could this evidence be used within my practice arena?

What benefits will the implementation of this evidence have for patients/carers/other healthcare workers?

What risks are associated with implementing this evidence?

What risks are associated with not implementing this evidence?

What are the opportunities for and constraints to implementing this evidence?

In this chapter you have read about the main methods for data collection and analysis, together with techniques for ensuring rigour in research studies. Using these approaches correctly, within the designs discussed in Chapter 6, will help you to find answers to your research questions. In addition, you can use this information to help you to assess the quality of other people's research before you consider implementing it in practice.

## ▦ Further reading

Atkinson I. Descriptive statistics. In: R Watson, H McKenna, S Cowman, J Keady (eds). *Nursing Research: Designs and methods.* 2008; Edinburgh: Churchill Livingstone.

Bannigan K, Watson R. Reliability and validity in a nutshell. *Journal of Clinical Nursing.* 2009; **18**(23): 3237–3243.

Clegg F. *Simple Statistics.* 1983; Cambridge: Cambridge University Press.

Mulhall A. In the field: notes on observation in qualitative research. *Journal of Advanced Nursing.* 2008; **41**(3): 306–313.

Nolan M. Qualitative data analysis: achieving order out of chaos. In: R Watson, H McKenna, S Cowman, J Keady (eds). *Nursing Research: Designs and methods.* 2008; Edinburgh: Churchill Livingstone.

Watson R. Inferential statistics. In: R Watson, H McKenna, S Cowman, J Keady (eds). *Nursing Research: Designs and methods.* 2008; Edinburgh: Churchill Livingstone.

## ▦ References

Bannigan K, Watson R. Reliability and validity in a nutshell. *Journal of Clinical Nursing.* 2009; **18**(23): 3237–3243.

Crabtree B, Miller W. *Doing Qualitative Research.* 1992; Thousand Oaks, CA: Sage Publications.

De Poy E, Gitlin L. *Introduction to Research. Understanding and Applying Multiple Strategies.* 1998; St Louis, MO: Mosby.

Denscombe M. *The Good Research Guide for Small Scale Social Research Projects.* 1998; Buckingham: Open University Press.

Dey I. *Qualitative Data Analysis.* 1993; London: Routledge.

le May A, Gabbay J. Evidence based practice in practice. In: G Lewith, J Cousins, H Walach (eds). *Clinical Research in Complementary Therapies.* 2011; Elsevier: Edinburgh.

Lowe D. *Planning for Medical Research: A practical guide to research methods.* 1993; Congleton: Astroglobe.

McDowell I, Newell C. *Measuring Health: A guide to rating scales and questionnaires.* Second edition. 1996; New York: Oxford University Press.

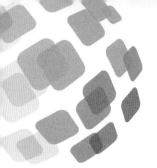

# Chapter 8

# Gaining permission for research

## ◼ Introduction

So you have an idea for research. Now you need permission to carry it out. Who you need permission from depends on the type of research you're planning as well as the type of participants involved. Research that involves the National Health Service (NHS) in any way must also consider the requirements of the Research Governance Framework (RGF) for Health and Social Care (DH 2005), which applies to all research involving:

- current or past NHS patients (including deceased), their relatives, NHS staff;
- data, organs or other tissue of past/present NHS patients;
- NHS premises or facilities;

and is intended to:

- safeguard participants and protect researchers;
- enhance ethical and scientific quality;
- minimize risk;
- monitor practice and performance;
- promote good practice and ensure that lessons are learned.

It defines the principles of 'good research' so that the public can have confidence in, and benefit from, health and social care research. Research that is not conducted in the NHS does not require Research Governance approval but all studies involving human participants need ethical approval and permission to access specific organizations and/ or samples – check with your organization as it may have specific requirements.

# Key principles of the RGF

The RGF sets out the core principles of good research governance, secured by key standards:

- *Ethics*: ensures participants' dignity, rights, safety and well-being, through independent ethical review, gaining informed consent, ensuring confidentiality and protection of data, consumer involvement and respect for diversity.
- *Science*: ensures that research design and methods are subject to independent expert review. If your project is part of a university course, systems will be in place for such review; if you work in the NHS, the research and development (R&D) office is likely to arrange it.
- *Information*: ensuring full and free access to information about research and its findings requires that they are publicly accessible; research that is not published is neither justifiable nor ethical.
- *Health and safety*: ensuring the safety of participants, researchers and other staff; demonstrated by understanding of, and adherence to, health and safety regulations.
- *Finance*: ensures financial probity and legal compliance in the conduct of research.
- *Employment*: ensuring that those undertaking research in the NHS hold substantive or honorary contracts and are insured for non-negligent harm. You may also need a Criminal Records Bureau check and/or occupational health screening.
- *Intellectual property*: concerns research outputs (e.g. inventions, knowledge, copyright) requiring that agreement is reached about who will be credited with authorship of papers or other intellectual property arising from research.

Guidance relating to research management and approval is subject to constant review and change; we must be up to date and adhere to its requirements.

# Seeking permission for research under the RGF (Figure 8.1)

As the RGF distinguishes between 'research', 'audit' and 'evaluation', you must first consider whether governance and ethical approval are needed (see Table 8.1). If it's research, register your project for research governance in relevant NHS organizations and submit the necessary paperwork; even if it is not research, you may still need permission to conduct your study – contact your R&D office to see if this applies to you.

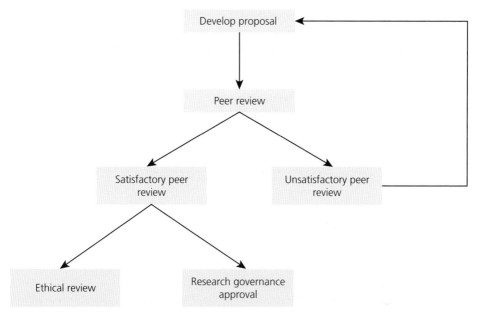

**Figure 8.1**  Summary: Research Governance Process

**Table 8.1**  Distinction between research, audit and evaluation (adapted from the National Patient Safety Agency 2011)

|  | Research | Audit | Evaluation |
|---|---|---|---|
| **Intent[1]** | To derive new knowledge and 'find out what we should be doing' | Measure level of care and 'find out if we are doing what we should be doing' | Measure level of care |
| **Treatment** | To study a treatment or intervention | Does not use a treatment without the firm support of clinicians | Does not use a treatment without the firm support of clinicians |
| **Allocation** | Treatment allocated by protocol | Treatment decisions made by clinicians and patients | Treatment decisions made by clinicians and patients |
| **Randomization** | If a study uses randomization it is a research study | Does not use randomization | Does not use randomization |

[1] Some projects may have more than one intent (purpose); in such cases, judgement is needed to establish the primary aim.

Approval is generally needed from two sources:

- ethical approval from an NHS or social care Research Ethics Committee (REC);
- research governance approval from an NHS Trust or primary care organization.

These requirements apply across the UK and you can apply for both using the Integrated Research Application System (IRAS) (**www.nres.npsa.nhs.uk**), coordinated by the National Research Ethics Service (NRES); it will be taken over by the Health Research Authority in the future (see Box 8.1).

---

**Box 8.1    The National Research Ethics Service**

The National Research Ethics Service has two functions, which are:

- to protect the rights, safety, dignity and well-being of research participants; and
- to facilitate and promote ethical research of potential benefit to participants, science and society.

The Integrated Research Application System:

- is a single system for applying for permission and approval for health and social care and community care research in the UK;
- allows you to enter information about your project once instead of duplicating information in separate application forms;
- uses filters to ensure that data collection is appropriate to the type of study and the permissions and approvals required;
- helps you meet regulatory and governance requirements.

**www.nres.npsa.nhs.uk**

---

Research governance approval will not be given unless ethical approval is gained. Despite common application procedures, ethics approval is provided by NHS or Social Care RECs and research governance by NHS organizations. The process takes time and effort; you must allow several months to prepare and gain ethics and research governance approval.

## ■ The first step

Before you can gain approval, you must write a proposal showing that your research is worthwhile and can be conducted competently and ethically; it must provide enough information to enable evaluation of your study (see Table 8.2).

---

**Exercise 8.1  A research proposal**

List what you think should be included in a research proposal. Now compare your responses to Table 8.2. Have you covered everything?

---

Your proposal must demonstrate that the research is important and that you have a good grasp of the relevant literature and major issues. Describe the research aims and methods (i.e. what you plan to do, why and how you're going to do it). Justify why you've chosen these methods and how they will answer the research question(s). Outline and address the ethical implications, the intended benefits of the study and how findings will be used/disseminated.

**Table 8.2** Outline of a research proposal

| |
|---|
| **Introduction:** Broad foundation of the problem leading to the study. |
| **Review of the literature:** Provides the background and context for the study, establishes the need for research and indicates your knowledge of the area. |
| **Purpose and rationale for the study:** Overall purpose; defines the specific area of the research and identifies specific research questions/hypotheses. Shows how your research will refine or extend existing knowledge. |
| **Design: methods and procedures:** Provides a rationale for your decision to use the selected methodology and analyses and describes the activities to be undertaken in detail. |
| Indicates the steps to be taken in answering the question(s) or testing the hypothesis/es. |
| Consideration of sampling, surveys, scales, interview protocols, questionnaires. |
| Overall plan for data collection and expected time schedule. |
| Outline of data analysis and any analytical tools you expect to use (e.g. ethnograph, NVIVO, SPSS). |
| **Ethical considerations.** |
| **The benefits of the work.** |
| **How the findings will be used and disseminated.** |
| **References:** List all the references cited in the text. |
| **Appendices:** Include copies of any instruments to be used or interview protocols to be followed. |
| Include Participant Information Sheet (see Table 8.3) and a consent form. |

# Ethical issues

Research ethics are central to all research involving human participants and, as nurses may be involved in research in many different ways (e.g. conducting research, collecting data for others, participating in research), they must understand the underlying ethical principles. Ask yourself the following questions about your work:

1. Does it involve people who are vulnerable or unable to give informed consent (e.g. children, people with learning disabilities) or in unequal relationships (e.g. prisoners)?

2. Is help needed from a gatekeeper to access participants (e.g. medical consultant, nursing home manager, nurse/midwife)?

3. Will people need to participate without their knowledge or consent (e.g. covert observation)?

4. Will it use any form of deliberate deception (excluding random allocation)?

5. Will it involve discussion of sensitive topics (e.g. sexual activity, drug use)?

6. Will it involve administration of drugs, placebos or other substances?

7. Does it involve invasive procedures (e.g. blood taking)?

8. Is it likely to cause stress, anxiety, pain or more than mild discomfort or cause harm or negative consequences beyond the risks encountered in normal life?

9. Will it involve prolonged or repetitive testing?

10. Will it involve offering participants financial or other inducement (other than reasonable expenses and compensation for time)?

11. Will it involve recruitment of patients or staff through the NHS?

If you have answered 'yes' to any of these questions, you will need ethical approval. Even if you have answered 'no', it's worth checking with someone in authority to ensure that your project can go ahead.

---

### Exercise 8.2  Ethical principles

What ethical principles do you believe are important in research? Compare your list with the material below.

---

## Ethical principles

Research ethics concerns the principles aimed at ensuring the rights, safety and well-being of participants which are underpinned by respect for human dignity protecting individual interests and integrity and guiding research planning and conduct. An overview is provided here; for further information see Beauchamp and Childress (2001).

**Autonomy,** the right of individuals to determine their own course of action and make judgements/decisions for themselves, underlies the need for informed consent. It also concerns the possibility that researchers might exert inappropriate power over participants (coercion) (Pink 2007). It's important that participants don't feel pressured (coerced) to take part (e.g. patients may worry about saying no or feel obliged to participate).

**Informed consent** comprises three elements – information, voluntariness and comprehension – and must be obtained before recruiting participants who must be given sufficient information about the study, the procedures involved and potential risks and benefits to ensure that they don't feel deceived or exploited. Information must be clear, straightforward and honest, explaining why the study is needed and what is required from participants. It should be provided verbally and in writing and potential participants must be allowed at least 24 hours to consider their involvement and ask questions. They should give their consent voluntarily and understand that they have the right to withdraw without prejudice and with no impact on their care. **Truth** (veracity) is, therefore, important; without this, participants can't exert their rights to informed consent, justice or fairness. You must show how you will meet these requirements and prepare a Participant Information Sheet (see Table 8.3) and consent form. However, people often don't, or can't, read an information sheet, so be prepared to talk this through, particularly when involving vulnerable people.

**Table 8.3** Information that must be included in a Participant Information Sheet (PIS)

- Purpose of the PIS.
- Duration and nature of the research.
- University, department, principal investigator and who is conducting the research and collecting the data; contact address and telephone number.
- Clear statement of exactly what participants are required to do (e.g. complete questionnaire, take part in focus groups, etc.) or what will happen to them.
- Description of possible advantages, benefits, disadvantages or risks of taking part. Include 'costs' involved in taking part in the study, including time involved.
- Description of any possible discomfort or inconvenience involved; procedures to be followed should adverse effects arise.
- Statement on the right to withdraw at any time without penalty or effect on treatment/care delivery.
- Procedures to protect participants from harm during the research and to assure confidentiality and anonymity.
- Information regarding the storage of data (security measures, length of time, etc.).
- How the results will be disseminated.
- Who to contact in case of questions or complaint.

The term 'vulnerable people' refers to many different groups (e.g. those with mental illness, learning disability or communication difficulties, prisoners). Their involvement in research raises problems that largely reflect the power imbalance between researchers and participants who may have difficulty in understanding what research is about, what their role will be or how its findings will be used. As it may be difficult for them to make their wishes and preferences known, they are entitled to special protection against abuse, discrimination and exploitation. You must develop appropriate strategies for communicating the implications of participating in research and, as some vulnerable people find being asked to sign a consent form worrying, consider ways of obtaining legitimate verbal consent.

When adults lack the mental capacity to make a fully informed decision, the Mental Capacity Act (DH 2005) applies in England and Wales. Research falling under the Act in England must be approved by an 'appropriate body', known as a 'flagged' NHS REC or approved social care REC; you will need specialist guidance, such as that provided by the NRES (**www.nres.npsa.nhs.uk**). In Scotland, such research falls under the Adults with Incapacity (Scotland) Act (2000); applications must be submitted to the Multicentre Research Ethics Committee (MREC) for Scotland.

Where research involves children under the age of 16 years, the requirements of the Children Act (1989) for England, and 1985 for Scotland, apply. Consent must be obtained from parents or those acting in *loco parentis* as it is assumed that children lack adequate decision-making capacity and their limited autonomy makes it impossible to obtain meaningful informed consent (Erb *et al* 2002). However, there is growing recognition that children have a right to participate in matters affecting their lives (Coyne and Gallagher 2011) and should be actively engaged wherever possible. They have the right to receive information, be listened to, have their wishes and feelings taken into account, and give or withhold consent if judged competent to do so (United Nations Convention on the Rights of the Child 1989). This protects their rights to self-determination, yet privileges respect for parents' rights in decision making concerning their child (Erb *et al* 2002). Thus, it is appropriate to seek consent from both parents and children themselves; if consent is gained from a relevant adult but the child clearly withholds consent or is distressed, the wishes of the child should prevail. Enabling children to engage in research requires practical considerations, such as preparing 'child-friendly' information sheets and consent forms.

Everyone is entitled to **privacy and confidentiality**, both on ethical grounds and under the Data Protection Act (1998); respecting this demonstrates respect for autonomy. People have the right to decide the time, extent and circumstances under which they will share or withhold information. This means not sharing personal details (that could identify individuals, families, activities or beliefs). As researchers we have a moral obligation to ensure that personal data are kept confidential and legal responsibilities under the Data Protection Act (1998). This should be emphasized on the Participant Information Sheet.

Anonymity is preserved by coding data, using numbers/pseudonyms, so that participants can't be identified in any presentation of the findings, and keeping personal information separate from the data. If you want to use photographs or excerpts from video recordings, written permission should be obtained after participants have reviewed the material.

Data protection also concerns the storage and retention of data, whether held manually or stored electronically. It must be physically secure (i.e. locked cupboard/cabinet for paper, visual or audio records). Electronically stored data must be password-protected; identifiable data must not be stored on laptop computers or pen/flash drives. Back-up media (e.g. CDs/DVDs) must also be password-protected.

In health and social care, data are usually stored for up to five years, but some organizations have different requirements, so check with your R&D office. Participants must be aware how long data will be retained and assured that their data will be secure.

**Justice** concerns the distribution of benefits and burdens of research requiring that standards and procedures for review are in place, ethics review is fair and transparent, participants are treated fairly, no person/group is discriminated against, and everyone is treated in a way that is morally right, without making potentially prejudicial distinctions; no part of the population must be unfairly burdened with research, neglected or discriminated against.

The main ethical issue here focuses on the inclusion of different groups. This can be tricky if you're interested in a specific population (e.g. older women, ethnic minorities, children), but it's important to show that you have thought about it and include it in your application.

It can never be guaranteed that research involving human participants won't cause harm. This includes more than physical harm and may describe emotional harm, upset or reputational damage. While many projects involve only minimal risk, others carry more substantial possibilities. You must demonstrate awareness of the risks and how they will be overcome.

The aim of research is to investigate 'something' designed to benefit future patients rather than those directly involved. The principle of **beneficence** imposes a duty to benefit others and maximize net benefits. Thus research must be intended to generate knowledge to produce benefits for participants, other individuals or wider society. Foreseeable harms must not outweigh anticipated benefits, thus addressing participants' welfare and rights and the ethical justification(s) for research.

In practice, this means that participants must not be subjected to unnecessary risks (**non-malificence**, do no harm). Their inclusion must be essential to achieving scientific or socially important aims that can't be achieved in any other way; research must involve the smallest number of people and tests to ensure scientifically valid data. RECs want to see that any risks to participants are balanced by potential benefits and that everything possible is done to offset them. For example, it's often believed that interviews don't carry any risk, but if the topic is sensitive or embarrassing, this may upset some people. You must show that you've considered this and that suitable arrangements are in place to support those needing further support after the interview (e.g. contact details for a counselling service).

## Ethics in research design

The research question(s) and/or hypothesis/es determine research design and approaches to data collection; justifying these and protecting participants' rights needs thought. All research raises some ethical questions and you must demonstrate how you will address them. Explain:

1. the rationale and the contribution that you believe the research will make; how the selected design/methodology achieves this;

2. how/if you've involved users in developing the project;

3. how the composition and size of the sample are justified;

4. how you will approach and recruit participants;

5. how you will gain informed consent, particularly from vulnerable people and those whose native language is not that in which the research is being conducted;

6. how you will ensure that participants don't feel pressurized/coerced to participate.

Care is needed when approaching participants through a 'gatekeeper' as they may be motivated by trust in the caregiver rather than by assessing the benefits and harms of participation.

Sample selection also raises ethical questions: who do you include or exclude? As sample size can significantly affect the meaning that can be attributed to the findings, you must justify this, showing that it will provide valid results. Where research is designed to enhance understanding, as in qualitative studies, this must be explained. Think carefully about your sample to determine which ethics committee you must go to – for example, if you include particular populations (e.g. vulnerable adults), additional requirements must be addressed.

## ■ Preparing to get permission

Once your proposal is complete and has been independently reviewed, you must negotiate access to your sample and gain written permission from managers and/or consultants to establish what you may and may not do during the study. If your plans change you must make them aware of this and get permission for the change(s).

Then decide where you need to submit your application and/or whether it is suitable for 'proportionate review' (see page 101). Studies involving any of the categories shown in Box 8.2 always require full REC review and must be submitted directly through the NRES and are allocated to an REC by the central allocation system. All research taking place on a single site is submitted directly to the local REC. This is likely to apply to most nursing research – contact your R&D office for advice.

| Box 8.2 | REC review |
| --- | --- |

The following types of application always require full REC review:

- Clinical trials of investigatory medicinal products or medical devices
- Research subject to the Mental Capacity Act (2005), or Adults with Incapacity (Scotland) Act (2000), or involving children, other vulnerable groups or prisoners
- Invasive basic science studies involving healthy volunteers
- Research involving exposure to ionizing radiation over and above that received in routine clinical care
- Gene therapy or a human tissue bank application
- Studies funded by the US Department of Health and Human Sciences
- Applications involving more than one site in England, health board in Scotland, regional office in Wales or anywhere in Northern Ireland

Now complete the NRES application forms using the online system (**www.nres.npsa.nhs.uk**). You must first register following the instructions given and using the available help and guidance. The form will filter unnecessary questions. Once the filter questions are complete, only questions relevant to your work will be asked.

Ensure you answer the questions asked and that your answers are consistent with your proposal. Keep the language simple – where you are asked for lay language, use it. Don't try to impress the REC by using academic or clinical jargon as not all members are either academics or clinicians. You must also submit additional documents such as the PIS (see Table 8.3, page 97), consent form(s), interview schedules, questionnaires, covering letters and recruitment advertisements or posters.

## Participant Information Sheets

Participants must take part freely and with adequate information and understanding; the PIS helps to ensure this. Think carefully about your participants' needs, making sure that the language is appropriate. You may need to prepare 'child-friendly' information sheets and consent forms, for example, or, in Wales, prepare information sheets in both English and Welsh (Welsh Language Act 1993). Guidance is available on the NRES website.

### Exercise 8.3 Design a PIS

Design a PIS for a study in which you're interested, then check with Table 8.3, page 97, and NRES guidance. Have you included all that is needed? Is the language appropriate to your audience? Now prepare a child-friendly version of the same information sheet.

Lastly, you will need other supplementary documentation such as letters from your sponsor and funding body (if appropriate) and copies of any independent reviews (this may have been arranged by your R&D office or university).

Don't be confused by the jargon surrounding 'sponsorship' – this doesn't refer to project funding as you might expect but to the organization guaranteeing the quality of the research and the competence of the researcher. While responsibility for the safe conduct of research lies with researchers, employers or, for students, universities, the REC must ensure that quality monitoring mechanisms are in place. Finally, a statement of indemnity is required from that organization. The need to provide these documents shows the importance of liaising with the R&D department early in the course of your work.

Once the documentation is complete, contact the REC administrator to obtain a unique study number and enter this onto the form before processing it both online and on hard copy.

## Proportionate review

Proportionate review (PR) is appropriate for studies presenting no material ethical issues (i.e. minimal risk, burden or intrusion for participants), enabling them to be rapidly reviewed (within 14 days of receipt) by a Proportionate Review Subcommittee (PRSC) on behalf of the REC. There are currently six such REC centres in England (London, East of England, South West, East Midlands, North East, North West), one in Wales and one in Scotland. Researchers don't have to be based in these regions and appropriate studies can be reviewed by any PRSC meeting.

The latest version of the NRES application form enquires whether an application is suitable for proportionate review (Question A6-3); guidance is available on the website (**www.nres.npsa.nhs.uk/applications/proportionate-review**). If you think this is appropriate, you can request that it be considered for PR. Staff who book in applications may also identify applications that may be suitable for PR. For your application to be suitable, the research must fit one of the categories listed in the No Material Ethical Issues Tool (NMEIT) (**www.nres.npsa.nhs.uk**) (see Box 8.3).

---

**Box 8.3    Proportionate review**

Types of research that may be suitable for proportionate review:

- Research using data or tissue that is anonymous to the researcher

- Studies using existing tissue samples already taken with consent for research

- Research using 'extra tissue' (e.g. blood taken at time of routine sampling or tissue taken at 'clinically directed' surgery) with permission for research

- Questionnaires, interviews or focus groups that don't include highly sensitive areas or where accidental disclosure wouldn't have serious consequences

- Research surveying the safety or efficacy of established non-drug treatments, involving limited intervention and no change to patients' treatment

Research involving children may be considered when it meets the above criteria.

---

If you think your study is suitable, contact your local REC office where the staff will ask a number of questions to ensure this is so before arranging for the study to be considered at the next available PRSC meeting. Unlike applications to the full committee, researchers are not required to attend the meeting; they may, however, be contacted (by phone or email) by an REC member if any clarification is required – this will be detailed in the validation letter from the REC office.

# ■ Conclusion

Anyone wanting to conduct research in the NHS must obtain REC and research governance approval. If this is part of a university course, check their ethics and governance approval processes; these will not supersede NHS requirements, however. This may seem daunting to novice researchers, but if enough time is allowed, and appropriate help and advice sought, it can be a straightforward process.

## Further guidance

Guidance for involving people with mental illness in research is available at: www.mrc.ac.uk/Utilities/Documentrecord/index.htm?d=MRC002409.

Guidance relating to involving children in research is available at: ethics.grad.ucl.ac.uk/forms/guidance1.pdf.

## References

Beauchamp TL, Childress JF. *Principles of Biomedical Ethics*. Fifth edition. 2001; Oxford: Oxford University Press.

Coyne I, Gallagher P. Participation in communication and decision-making: children and young people's experiences in hospital. *Journal of Clinical Nursing*. 2011; **20**: 2334–2345.

Department of Health. *Mental Capacity Act*. 2005; London: Department of Health. Chapter 9. Also available at **www.opsi.gov.uk/ACTS/acts2005/ukpga_20050009_en_1**.

Department of Health. *Research Governance Framework for Health and Social Care*. Second edition. 2005; London: The Stationery Office.

Erb TO, Schulman SR, Sugarman J. Permission and assent for clinical research in pediatric anesthesia. *Anesthesia and Analgesia*. 2002; **94**(5): 1155–1160.

National Patient Safety Agency 2011. **www.nres.npsa.nhs.uk/**.

Pink S. *Doing Visual Ethnography*. Second edition. 2007; London: Sage Publications. pp40–62.

The Scottish Government. *Adults with Incapacity Act 2000*. Edinburgh.

United Nations. *Convention on the Rights of the Child*. 1989; Geneva: United Nations.

*Welsh Language Act 1993*. London: The Stationery Office.

## Chapter 9

# Telling people about your research

## ◼ Introduction

We must share the knowledge gained through research if it is to influence practice or policy. There is little point in conducting a study if we don't tell others what we've found and how our findings contribute to nursing knowledge and practice (Byrne 2001). Thus, dissemination is central to research and helps practitioners to access information about proposed interventions and to improve patient outcomes (Scott and McSherry 2009). It needs careful thought and planning. This chapter considers the approaches we can use to disseminate our work.

> **Exercise 9.1  Disseminating research results**
>
> What is the purpose of disseminating research results? What factors should you take into account when developing a dissemination plan?

## ◼ Dissemination

All dissemination should have a purpose, such as to:

- raise awareness of your work;
- communicate with the widest possible audience;
- target specific audiences who will benefit from the results;
- help to get feedback on your work, to promote it and yourself and 'sell' your outputs.

### Issues to consider

What do you want to achieve: describe your research, highlight your finding(s), get feedback? Think about people/organizations that might benefit from and/or use your research. Could they help you to reach your target audience? Identify any formal and informal networks, influential professionals or trusted opinion leaders you could approach who might influence users through their credibility and expertise.

Next, consider how to disseminate your work. This may involve communicating your findings to those working where the study was conducted, through reports and/or presentations, speaking/writing at a local, regional, national or international level, or interacting with policy makers and healthcare audiences to facilitate its uptake in practice. Ask yourself:

- Who are my target audience? How can I reach them most effectively?
- What methods can I use?
- Could others help me to communicate with users? How can I contact them?

Effective dissemination often relies on a combination of approaches to reach the widest possible audience in ways that are accessible and easy to use.

## ◼ Writing for publication

Writing is important in communicating knowledge, skills and experience to the wider nursing population (Meadows 2004). You may need to prepare a report for a funding body or for the organization where you work or choose to write for publication. Though the thought may be horrifying, it is not, in practice, very different from the writing you do at university. There is nothing inherently mysterious about it – what distinguishes authors from novices is that they understand that good writing requires sustained effort (Stepanski 2002) and lots of practice.

Though publishing contributes to debate or adds to the body of knowledge, researchers write for many other reasons, including personal satisfaction/development, strengthening their CV and advancing their career. However, barriers, obstacles or excuses often stop them writing – the most common are lack of confidence, fear of criticism/rejection, being 'too busy' or not knowing where to start. The only way to overcome these is to start writing.

> **Exercise 9.2  Barriers to writing**
>
> Take time to identify your personal barriers to writing. How can you overcome them?

### *Getting started*

Before you begin, think about:

- who you want to read your paper and why they will be interested in your work;
- what is the most important thing you want them to take from your paper;
- what you want them to do as a result of reading your paper.

Readers will want to know why you did the work, how you did it (methods), the results (findings) and your interpretation of them, the conclusions you've drawn and their relevance to practice. Knowing your audience and what they're likely to want helps you to plan your paper.

Targeting a paper to a particular journal is '*the* most important factor in successful writing for publication' (Cook 2000), so think carefully about the available journals. This may be relatively simple when there are few journals in your field but more complex when a number could be appropriate. Consider both the type of journal and what is most suitable – a scholarly or academic journal is appropriate for an empirical research paper, but you may also want to consider a subject-specific journal or professional magazine with a wider circulation. Taking time to identify the 'right' journal which offers the best possibility of publication is important (see Table 9.1).

**Table 9.1**  Questions to ask when choosing a journal

- What is its purpose?
- What regular features does it include?
- What topics and articles have been recently published?
- What elements and features do the articles include?
- How long are the articles?
- How deep is the information?
- How formal or informal are the design, writing and graphics?
- Is your paper relevant to the journal's content?

---

**Exercise 9.3  Journals**

Select two or three journals that you're interested in, look at the contents of each edition over the last two years and consider the following:

a. Check the purpose, aims and scope. Is your intended paper appropriate?

b. Identify what they have previously published on your topic.

c. Read some of the papers. Look at the format, style, voice and intended audience.

d. Consider whether there are gaps in the literature that your paper might fill.

e. Obtain author guidelines to establish the journal's expectations.

## ■ Preparing your manuscript

Having made your decision, read and follow the guidelines which specify how to present manuscripts and what they should contain (see Table 9.2). Don't take them lightly – manuscripts may be rejected out of hand if you don't follow them. They will include factors such as the:

- required structure;
- style of the abstract;
- maximum word number;
- number of key words: choose carefully – they help people find your paper;
- number of tables and/or figures allowed;
- how references should be presented;
- the required line spacing and page margins;
- details of how to submit your paper.

Some journals also require you to outline what is already known about the topic and what your paper contributes to that knowledge.

**Table 9.2** General structure of a paper

| Introduction: | Sets the context and states the problem to be investigated. |
|---|---|
| Literature review: | A critical evaluation of the current literature on the topic (i.e. why the work was needed). |
| Method: | How the study was carried out. |
| Results: | What was found? |
| Discussion: | What the findings show. |
| Conclusion: | Importance of the findings and their relevance to practice/service delivery/ policy. |

## Planning

It is common to overlook the need for planning. This is a mistake! Time spent thinking about the purpose and key messages is never wasted – it helps you to think clearly about your topic and saves time in the long run. There is no single way of doing this. Use whatever tools you find helpful: index cards, diagrams, concept maps or simple outline.

Begin by writing statements to help keep you focused. For example, summarize the key message(s) in a few sentences; focus on what you want readers to know and what you want them to do with the information. Keep these in mind as you write. Now look at the headings required and identify the points for inclusion in each section. This is the outline of your paper.

## Starting to write

Don't waste time thinking about a great title or opening line. Instead start with the part you feel most confident about, even if it's in the middle – you'll feel much better when you have written 'something'. Work through your outline, writing notes about each area. Don't worry about the quality of the writing – this comes later. Returning to the title and introductory paragraph(s) is easier when your paper is outlined.

Now, work through your notes, succinctly explaining the background to the study, showing why the work was necessary and what would be gained if the question was answered or the problem solved. Describe how this was investigated and what you found. Discuss your findings in the context of the literature and draw conclusions about them, their implications and relevance to practice/policy. Put your draft away for a few days – you'll return to it fresh and see it more critically.

## Basic elements of good writing

The foundations of good writing are clarity, simplicity and accuracy, so try to choose the simplest and most accurate word to express ideas and make your meaning clear (see Table 9.3). You do not need to use long words or 'jargon' to impress others; it's better to use words that are simple and easily understood (e.g. 'use' rather than 'utilize', 'make sure of' instead of 'ascertain'). Be precise and say what you mean. Define key terms and concepts in the introduction and use the same term consistently throughout – without this, readers may become confused, thus detracting from your key message(s).

**Table 9.3** Tips for writing a paper

- Use short words where possible.
- Use language and terms that will be readily understood.
- Avoid jargon – use simple language, taking care to explain difficult concepts or terminology.
- Avoid unnecessary repetition.
- Explain abbreviations the first time you use them.
- Maintain confidentiality.
- Reduce complex phrases.
- Remove redundant words.
- Emphasize the relevance of your paper to the wider community.
- Remember that 'less is more' (i.e. shorter is better) (brevity).

Good writing is also carefully structured, containing sentences that are clear, direct and brief. A sentence is a group of words about a single idea containing at least one subject and one verb. The subject, the focus of the sentence, should appear early; this is a noun whereas verbs are 'action' or 'doing' words (Zeiger 2000). In the example 'Nurses provide care for patients', the noun is 'nurses' and the verb is 'provide'.

A paragraph is a group of related sentences exploring and developing a single idea. It should be unified and coherent. Each sentence should focus on the topic and the relationship between sentences must show development of the idea. Paragraphs usually comprise at least three sentences, and often more. Though there is no limit on the number of sentences in individual paragraphs, brevity is valuable and reduces the potential for confusion. While it's common to write as we think or speak, this rarely 'translates' into good writing; instead it will be confusing and difficult to read. Be disciplined and self-critical.

### Exercise 9.4  Writing practice

Try writing a paragraph – using clear and simple sentences – to explain an aspect of nursing care or a patient's condition. Put this away for a few days and then look at it again. Does it explain the key ideas clearly and concisely? When you're satisfied with it, ask some friends or colleagues to look at it and comment on these aspects.

Exercise 9.4 will probably show you that, after completing the first draft, you will need to simplify what you've written and remove unnecessary words, sentences, even paragraphs. You may need to rewrite sentences and/or paragraphs to enhance their clarity and brevity. Expect to rewrite your material several times – we all do!

Ensure that your text is grammatically correct, your ideas are presented clearly and key concepts/terms are explained and used consistently. Are your methods explained so that it's clear how data were collected and analysed? Is your discussion logical? Does it include statements of the main findings and the strengths and weaknesses of your work in relation to other studies? Are the meaning(s) of your study, its impact and implications clear? Have you identified unanswered questions and areas for future research? Finally, are your conclusions justified by the results you've presented? If so, write your abstract, a succinct summary, following the guidelines, and make sure it is within the word limit.

Check that your references are complete and that you haven't plagiarized anyone's work. Plagiarism, the act of presenting the material, ideas and arguments of another person(s) using their words as if they were your own, may deceive readers about their source. Paraphrasing, in ways that can deceive readers, is also plagiarism. Ensure that other people's words, if used directly, are presented using quotation marks and attributing the source (Price 2010).

### Exercise 9.5  Tidying up

Once your paper is complete, read it out loud to see whether it's clear or whether you need to remove unnecessary words/sentences. Do you need to clarify or simplify the language or its meaning or remove jargon?

If some of the material is complex or difficult to understand, would it be clearer in tables or diagrams (see Table 9.4)? Finally, review its accuracy and appearance. Once you're happy, print it out and ask colleagues/friends to read it and offer advice. A paper is well written if someone who is not involved can read and understand it, so ask them to identify areas that are unclear. Use their advice to improve your paper – after all, you want to produce the best paper that you can.

**Table 9.4** Principles of good tabulation

| |
|---|
| 1. Tables need a short explanatory title. |
| 2. Units of measurement must be clear and, if necessary, defined in a footnote. Every column/row should have clear heading. |
| 3. Use different rulings to break up larger tables to make them easier to understand. |
| 4. When useful, insert both column and row totals. |
| 5. Consider whether two or three simple tables may be better than one large and cumbersome table. |
| 6. Be clear what you want the table to show. Remember that it's easier to absorb figures from columns rather than rows. |
| 7. Tables should be self-explanatory and summarize relevant data. |

## *Finalizing and submitting your paper*

Ensure the paper is formatted according to the guidelines and includes appropriate figures (pictures/diagrams) and tables if needed. Remember that you must submit the final version: you can't make any changes after acceptance, though you can correct spelling mistakes or misprints. Once you're satisfied, establish how the journal wants papers submitted (for most this will be electronically). Submit your paper!

Do not submit work to several journals simultaneously. If your paper is rejected you can submit to another journal, but you must approach only one at a time due to copyright and publishing rights agreements. Of course, if submitting elsewhere, you may have to modify the paper to match that journal's requirements.

Most journals will send your manuscript to at least two referees who will examine your work critically, comparing it with the expected standard. If necessary, they will comment on issues that need to be addressed to bring your paper up to that standard. This can be disappointing, particularly if it's your first paper, but it happens to all of us. Remember, their job is to ensure that only the best papers are published.

Read the referee's comments carefully and respond to them before returning a revised manuscript. This can be useful: you're getting free advice from experts. You may not agree with them, but if you don't, explain why, justifying this with clear arguments. Editors want to make sure that only high-quality work is published. What is required will be explained in a detailed letter specifying the changes needed. If you're unclear then contact the editor and ask for clarification.

## ■ Conferences

Presenting conference papers offers opportunities to share knowledge, develop communication skills, help raise your profile as a researcher and get immediate feedback. However, the time allocated to a paper may be short and opportunities to reach a multi-disciplinary audience limited and, if there are parallel or concurrent sessions, the audience may be small.

## *Things to consider*

Presenting for the first time is daunting but is made easier by good planning and preparation. Think carefully about what you want to achieve by your presentation and who you want to present it to as you can do this at many different levels, including local study days, before attempting a national or international event.

If you want to gain experience of presenting in a relatively safe environment, choose a local study day; if, however, you want to gain prestige and disseminate your work more widely, choose a higher-profile event (i.e. national/international conference). Both offer opportunities to network with colleagues sharing similar interests and the chance to influence practice and generate interest in your work.

Also consider the audience that a conference serves and address their interests. For example, if they are primarily researchers, you may want to emphasize methodological aspects of your work, but it may be better to focus on practical aspects for practitioners.

## *Where do I start?*

Think about what you want to say, why people need to know it, why they would care about it and what they would gain by knowing it. Also consider what you can present clearly and concisely in the time available, usually 15–30 minutes. This is unlikely to allow you to present the whole project, so you may want to discuss one element in-depth rather than attempt to cover everything in a rushed, sketchy way. Good presenters recognize this, tailor their presentation to fit and keep an eye on the time during the presentation.

## *Preparing your paper*

So, you've got something important to say and 15 minutes to say it? This needs careful thought. Good preparation is key. Don't think of it as 'writing' a paper, but instead outline your points and write as you speak. Imagine someone asking you about your topic and, in developing arguments and picking examples, listen to how you talk about them. You probably use shorter sentences and more colloquial language than when writing; this makes your paper lively and interesting.

You need to convince the audience that your paper is worth listening to, so start by telling them how you became interested in the topic or relate an anecdote from your research. People are more likely to pay attention and feel affinity with a speaker if they know something about them. Then move on to your key point(s).

Plan your paper so that the most interesting and important information is presented first and then build on it. In other words, 'Tell 'em what you're going to tell 'em, tell 'em, then tell 'em what you told 'em'! So outline your argument early, recap frequently and summarize clearly.

Signal the end with an appropriate slide saying something like 'So, what can we conclude from this?', conveying your current understanding and highlighting outstanding points for consideration. This is often where later conversations start – chatting about your work is important and can lead to new insights or collaborations.

Importantly, leave time for questions which offer a chance to elaborate on things that weren't clear or cover something that everyone wants to know but you forgot to say (see page 114).

## Using visual aids

There are many options for visual aids, but don't try to be too clever and don't go mad with PowerPoint. Slides are intended to help the audience, so make sure they communicate your point. For a 15–20-minute presentation, 6–12 slides are enough. Use them to present things that are difficult to describe (such as graphs and diagrams) or highlight key points, but don't just read what is on your slides – supplement them with anecdotes or summarize their content. Make sure that the audience can read them using a dark text on a light background, with no more than 10 lines per slide (20–30 point font).

## Rehearsing and giving the presentation

Rehearsing helps to clarify the amount of information that you can convey in the time allocated and allow time for questions. Practice also helps you to become familiar with the material so that when you perform 'for real', you aren't starting from scratch – this increases your confidence. Ask friends/colleagues to listen and comment on the paper (did they understand and enjoy it?) and your presentation (did you talk too fast? was it monotonous?).

Practice can also help you decide whether to read from your script or talk through your slides. The latter undoubtedly requires more confidence – you will need brief notes to guide you and indicate when to move on. If you decide to read from a script, print it in large font, making it easier to read – and find your place if you lose it.

On the day, remember this is a formal occasion and dress accordingly. While you don't need to wear a suit or dress, be smart. Arrive early, check out the room and ensure that any equipment you need is working and you know how to use it. Seek help if not. Then, when the time for your presentation arrives, take a deep breath, smile and walk to the lectern. To ensure you keep to time, put your watch on the lectern; although the chairperson will indicate when you're reaching the end, it is more professional to finish on time.

Start by making some informal comment – the weather, the room, the size of the audience – to help you feel in control. Remember, you have a good paper that people want to hear, take another deep breath and begin. Project your voice and look at the audience. Pick one or two people in different parts of the room and move your gaze between them; this will also engage others sitting nearby. If one responds with a smile, return to them as you develop your points. Further smiles will increase your confidence.

Speak up and speak slowly. Try to vary your tone and inflection – you want the audience to stay awake! When you reach particularly important points, give them extra emphasis or repeat them to ensure they're not lost. It's helpful to highlight things you want to emphasize on your notes.

If your timing begins to slip, don't rush through your slides in an attempt to catch up. Instead, make it clear that you are moving on to key slides or points. This suggests you're in control and helps retain the audience's respect.

When you've finished, ask for questions. Remember that the audience may want to learn more, clarify something or make a point of their own. You may be asked to expand or repeat something or engage in debate about something you said. People ask questions because they're interested and want to know more. Wait for a 'roving microphone' to reach them before accepting the question. It is good practice to repeat the question, allowing you to check the intended meaning. Don't be afraid to say you don't know or 'I hadn't thought about that – thank you for pointing it out'. Keep your answers relatively brief, allowing others to ask their questions.

Remember that everyone is nervous before giving a paper, even those who've done it for years. This is good and gets your adrenaline flowing. Try to relax, breathe deeply and enjoy the experience. It will be over before you know it!

## Posters

Posters offer a more informal means of presentation and the opportunity to discuss aspects of your work after the poster has been read (MacIntosh-Murray 2007). Combining text and graphics in posters offers a different way of communicating ideas and a chance for many people to see your work.

Posters are less formal than presentations and can be designed and organized well in advance. As the goal is to get the main points across to as many people as possible, posters must do the 'talking'. Consider them as a 'snapshot' of your work, providing a summary to encourage colleagues to want to learn more or engage in discussion. Your tasks are to convince them that your work is worthwhile, be available to answer questions and provide further details. A well-designed poster gives the audience a clear take-away message that can be grasped in the few minutes they spend reading it.

The best posters include material that can be presented visually (e.g. flow charts) (MacIntosh-Murray 2007) as such information is more easily assimilated. As they must be legible from a distance of 3–4 feet, use a minimum font size of 18–20 point. Plan the layout carefully. You will be told the space available, so mark out the appropriate space on a table or floor and do an initial layout to help you judge the detail you can include.

Don't try to jam every inch of your poster with graphics and text. Try different layouts until you're happy.

As most conferences include many posters, first impressions are important. The trick is to make yours stand out and attract attention. Select a 'good' title, treating this as a headline, keeping it short and sharp to 'sell' your work – it may be the first thing people see and should make them want to read more. Indicate the topic under discussion and ensure it is legible from at least 6 feet away.

Then, before starting to prepare your poster, consider what you want those viewing it to do. Engage in discussion? Learn enough to want to try something for themselves? Design your poster accordingly.

Many of the rules of writing also apply to posters. Identify your audience and provide the appropriate scope and depth of content. Provide a succinct summary of the background, hypothesis/es tested/question(s) answered, major results and conclusions. Remember, short, simple messages are more memorable.

Everything on the poster should help convey the message – don't try to give too much information. The text must be clear and concise. Use short, declarative sentences (statements) to explain the background, what you found and why it matters, but limit your methods to a few sentences – if someone wants to know more, they'll ask. Use arrows or numbers to guide them through the poster logically and ensure that the main points can be read at eye level.

Use accepted titles for sections (i.e. introduction (or background), methods, results, discussion, conclusions, references). Keep text to a minimum by using key words/phrases throughout.

Good illustrations can transform a mass of complex data into a coherent and convincing 'story'. A well-designed diagram, graph or table can say more than a thousand words and simplify complex material. Make these easy to interpret, perhaps using colour to indicate different categories in a table or using different styles to distinguish between lines on a graph. Clearly label any drawings and ensure that all illustrations are legible from a distance – drawings should be at least 8x10 inches.

Make sure that you include clear conclusions that are justified by the results and identify their implications and relevance to practice or policy.

Lastly, ensure that your poster is easy to read – leaving white space between the elements helps. Also use a consistent style throughout to maintain fluency and flow. This means that:

- headings should appear in the same position on all pages;
- graphs should be presented in the same size and scale, especially if they will be compared;
- either bold or italic lettering should be used for emphasis, and don't change between them;
- all figure and table captions are positioned in the same place relative to the material.

Remember that a poster should tell a 'story' about what you've done. Use colour to make it more attractive to the casual eye, thus tempting observers to look more closely. However, choose colours carefully and stick to two or three to stand out against your background. Dark colours generally look better against a light background than light colours against dark.

Make it easy for visitors to contact you later by clearly displaying your contact information. Let them read your poster at their own pace but be attentive and open and answer questions – this is your opportunity to get feedback on your work.

Occasionally, you may also be required to give a short 10–15-minute verbal presentation of the research and the principles of preparing a presentation will help.

## Summary

Dissemination is essentially about the transfer of knowledge that we have and want others to have. We therefore need to decide whether our work should be known by nurses working in a particular field, other researchers or those in management positions (Price 2010). This helps us to provide the audience with useful and relevant material.

Yet although dissemination is an important part of the research–practice continuum, it is increasingly recognized that the full potential for research evidence to improve practice in healthcare has not yet been realized (Wilson *et al* 2010). It is up to us to change this by telling others about our research through publications and/or conference presentations.

## References

Byrne M. Disseminating and presenting qualitative research findings. *AORN Journal*. 2001; **74**(5): 731–732.

Cook R. Knowing your journals. In: R Cook, A Norman. *The Writer's Manual: A step-by-step guide for nurses and other health professionals*. 2000; Abingdon: Radcliffe Medical Press. Chapter 3, pp23–34.

MacIntosh-Murray A. Poster presentations as a genre in knowledge communication: a case study of forms, norms and values. *Science Communication*. 2007; **28**(3): 347–376.

Meadows KA. So you want to do research? (6) Reporting research. *British Journal of Community Nursing*. 2004; **9**(1): 37–41.

Price B. Disseminating best practice through publication in journals. *Nursing Standard*. 2010; **24**(26): 35–41.

Scott K, McSherry R. Evidence-based nursing: clarifying the concepts for nurses in practice. *Journal of Clinical Nursing*. 2009; **18**(8): 1085–1095.

Stepanski LM. Becoming a nurse-writer: advice on writing for professional publication. *Journal of Infusion Nursing*. 2002; **25**(2): 134–140.

Wilson P, Pettigrew M, Calnan MW, Nazareth I. Disseminating research findings: what should researchers do? A systematic scoping review of conceptual frameworks. *Implementation Science.* 2010; **5**:91: doi:10.1186/1748-5908-5-91.

Zeiger M. Sentence structure. In: M Zeiger. *Essentials of Writing Biomedical Research Papers.* Second edition. 2000; New York: McGraw-Hill. pp22–50.

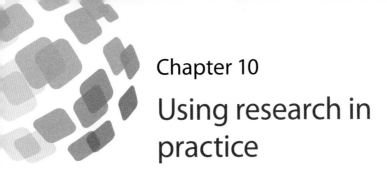

# Chapter 10

# Using research in practice

## ◼ Introduction

Every nurse needs to make every effort to use, as Cullum *et al* (2008 p2) put it, 'valid, relevant research-based information in (their) decision making' since delivering research-based care is central to achieving the best care. However, doing this is not as simple as it may first appear. This chapter will help you to start thinking about how you can use research in practice to provide better care. It starts by illustrating some of the barriers to using research that you might have to overcome and some of the opportunities for using research in practice that you might capitalize on. It then moves on to give an overview of some of the processes you might use to help you in implementing research.

## ◼ Barriers to the use of research evidence in practice

Over the past five years the UK government, the Higher Education Funding Council, the Department of Health and research funders have placed more emphasis on the need to increase the impact of research at 'the bedside' in order to improve patient care and justify their considerable financial investment in research. Despite an associated effort to make research more readily available, in guidelines and policy statements, many practitioners would agree that nursing decisions are still not always informed by the best and most up-to-date research. But why is this so? Numerous researchers have tried to answer this question, hoping that by identifying barriers to research use, they will be able to construct suitable interventions in order to promote better use of research. Let's take a look at what these barriers are.

Kajermo *et al* (2010) brought together data from 63 research studies that have used the BARRIERS scale to assess barriers to nurses' research use over the past 20 years. This systematic review concludes that the main barriers are related to the setting in which implementation occurs and the presentation of research findings. The authors state that barriers were consistent over time and also location. More extensive qualitative data from a study of practitioners' and managers' cultures of research (le May *et al* 1998) suggested that while some barriers do revolve around the setting in which nurses work, and the jargon used in the presentation of research findings (see Box 10.1), there are other important factors, such as attitudes, beliefs and professional relationships, that need to be considered.

| Box 10.1 | Practitioners' perceived barriers to research-based practice (adapted and updated from le May *et al* 1998) |
|---|---|

**Attitudes**

- Lack of cooperation
- Lack of motivation
- Fear
- Resistance to change
- Acceptance of ritualized or traditional practice

**Beliefs**

- Research will not make a difference
- Research data are not appropriate
- Conviction that current practice is OK

**Professional relationships**

- Medical staff block implementation
- Medical staff consider nursing research substandard
- Nursing colleagues are uncooperative
- Senior staff are resistant to change
- Low grading of research staff and often insecure posts

**Organizational issues**

- Time
- Pressure of workload
- Too much change

**Educational issues**

- Practitioners unaware of or unable to access research
- Lack of skills in critical appraisal
- Lack of skills in change management
- Research reports are jargonistic
- Implementing new research may mean developing different clinical skills

Furthermore, Gerrish *et al's* (2008) survey showed distinct differences between junior and senior nurses. While all 598 respondents said they were confident finding and using research evidence in practice, the senior nurses not only felt more confident accessing various sources of evidence (e.g. published sources and the internet) but were also confident in initiating change. Conversely, junior nurses were less confident about finding out about their organization and in implementing change. Lack of time and resources were also noted as major barriers by the more junior nurses but not by their senior colleagues, who felt able to overcome these limitations. Barriers cited by clinical nurse specialists in Canada (Profetto-McGrath *et al* 2007) support previous research and included lack of time, lack of resources and lack of receptivity at both clinical and organizational levels.

There seems, then, to be some consistency emerging in relation to the barriers identified, with nurses' use of research-based information being affected by several tangible challenges associated with:

- their work setting – lack of receptivity at clinical and organizational levels;
- the way research findings are presented;
- a lack of time;
- a lack of resources or the inappropriateness of available resources.

These may also be influenced by their attitudes and beliefs about research and their ability to implement change.

In addition to the barriers detailed above, practitioners sometimes suggest that the wrong research is being done as the results will not answer the questions to which they need answers. Increasingly, efforts are being made to minimize this mismatch by strengthening interactions between practitioners and researchers in order to fine-tune research questions and designs to meet the needs of practice.

## Encouraging the use of research evidence in practice

Knowing the barriers that nurses face in using research should make it easier to design interventions to help them. A quick literature search reveals that, over the past 20 years, many different approaches have been used to encourage nurses around the world to use research evidence in practice, with varying degrees of success. Given this huge literature, I looked for a systematic review in order to provide conclusive evidence of which approaches were best.

Thompson *et al's* (2007) systematic review is the only one to focus on interventions aimed at increasing research use in nursing. They took a highly structured approach, including only the most robust studies available. Although 8,000 titles were screened, only four studies met the inclusion criteria – three randomized controlled trials and one controlled before-and-after study. The principal intervention in all four studies was education, but it wasn't just simply providing education that mattered, it was the way that education was delivered that impacted on its success (or not). When education occurred in researcher-led educational meetings it was ineffective (two studies). However, when a local opinion leader led the meeting, it was effective (one study) and when the education occurred in multi-disciplinary committee meetings around a particular topic (oncology pain), it was also effective (one study). Unfortunately, the restrictive methodology of the systematic review has not got us much further forward other than to say that in some cases education works, while in others it doesn't. But it does suggest that education associated with an environment in which trusted colleagues are present (either as opinion leaders or as multi-disciplinary team co-workers) may make it more successful.

| Box 10.2 | Opportunities to develop research-based practice (adapted and updated from le May *et al* 1998) |
|---|---|

**Organizational support**

- Specific research and development strategy for Trust or for nursing
- Enhanced links with education providers
- Funding for courses and workshops; clinical academic career structures
- Specific appointments with an emphasis on research and practice/teaching
- Identification and support of champions for nursing

**New 'structures'**

- Research fora
- Research awareness groups
- Proactive research/ethics committees
- Research centres
- Nursing development units
- Collaborations for Leadership in Applied Health Research and Care (CLAHRC) funded by National Institute for Health Research (NIHR) at the Department of Health

**Inter-professional relationships**

- Multi-professional initiatives, e.g. guideline development
- Multi-disciplinary research: multi-agency research

**Changing individuals**

- Greater uptake of continuing education
- Recognition of importance of research by individuals
- Diploma and degree courses increasing individual skills and knowledge

Education was also an important feature for Profetto-McGrath *et al's* (2007) sample of clinical nurse specialists in Canada, along with peers and organizational support. Organizational support, inter-professional relationships and education also featured in le May *et al's* (1998) study of nurses and their managers in England. However, so did other interesting factors, namely reorganizations in the National Health Service (NHS) and the creation of new structures/fora (see Box 10.2).

In fact, several NHS reorganizations have occurred since this study (le May *et al* 1998) was completed, with the emergence of new structures that have offered many opportunities for the development of closer links between researchers and practitioners. Probably the most ambitious of these is the Collaborations for Leadership in Applied Health Research and Care (CLAHRC) initiative, developed in 2008 by the National Institute for Health Research (NIHR) at the Department of Health, in response to the Cooksey Report (2006). The CLAHRC's primary functions are to conduct high-quality applied health research, implement findings from research in clinical practice and increase the capacity of NHS organizations to engage with and apply research, including continuing professional development (**http://clahrc-sy.nihr.ac.uk/about.html**).

Alongside this, there has been the almost parallel development of structures within the NHS and the higher education sector that gave rise to the creation of formal Clinical Academic Career pathways (United Kingdom Clinical Research Collaboration (UKCRC) 2007). Another initiative spearheaded by the NIHR to promote closer links between research and practice, this encourages practitioners to stay in practice and develop their research skills, splitting their workload between delivering care and researching it. This supports the already established nursing and midwifery consultant posts which have the remit, although not as explicitly detailed, to link closely the implementation of research with providing care.

## ■ Frameworks for improving the use of research in practice

Several researchers, practitioners and academics have put forward models or frameworks which, if followed, might improve the use of research-based information in practice. Probably the best known of these are the models developed and refined over the past ten years by a team of researchers at the Royal College of Nursing in the UK – the Promoting Action on Research Implementation in Health Services (PARiHS) framework (Kitson *et al* 1998), two Canadian teams working to produce the Ottawa Model of Research Use (OMRU) (Logan and Graham 2010), the Knowledge-to-Action (KTA) framework (Graham and Tetroe 2010) and the Australian Joanna Briggs Institute (JBI).

| Box 10.3 | A consultant nurse's view |
|---|---|

What do the nurse implementing clinical research and Walt Disney have in common? Well, some of you may have your own version of the answer, but my response is, the 'Law of Doing the Impossible'! Walt Disney spoke about the importance of doing the impossible through using creativity and overcoming impossible situations with imaginative solutions. This is not unlike how nurses today work in challenging clinical situations and look for improved patient outcomes.

Clinical nurses are ideally placed to spot the difficult problems that patients, families and staff face in healthcare delivery. When did you last think at work, 'Why are we doing it this way?' Well, whatever that was, that's an idea for research right there. My clinical work focuses around supporting the chronically critically ill person in the intensive care unit (ICU) and those at end of life. I've often thought about what happens to bereaved families once they leave the ICU. And this has strongly influenced my research interviewing bereaved families in ICU to explore the impact of information and support given to them.

However, working with research comes in two parts. Once research has been undertaken, clinical nurses must then work to implement findings to make a difference to patients. As demonstrated in this chapter, this part of the research process is pivotal. It requires us all to convince, challenge and have conviction in our practice. Is this easy? No way! Is it necessary? You bet!

So what works for me? Know your facts and know how to deliver them with confidence in order to convince others. Know your audience and how best to talk with them. Learn how to present different arguments to diverse groups (doctors, nurses, physiotherapists), so you can challenge them to review and change their practice. Learn how to manage yourself when confronting others and know where your allies and adversaries are. Above all, have conviction in your practice. If you believe that implementing a research finding is important in practice and for patients, then drive that change through and embed it into your clinical area. Your enthusiasm will permeate even your most stalwart of objectors. As Walt Disney said, 'It's kind of fun to do the impossible!'

Maureen Coombs RN PhD
Consultant Nurse Critical Care/Senior Lecturer
Southampton University Hospitals Trust/University of Southampton

The main elements of these models are presented in Table 10.1, but further details of these and several other models and frameworks for implementing research into practice are presented in a comprehensive textbook edited by Rycroft-Malone and Bucknall (2010).

These models can appear a little esoteric to new students and practitioners, so you might find it helpful to start off with a simpler, more straightforward approach.

## A simple process to guide your implementation of research

As you read more widely you will come across a greater variety of processes through which research can be implemented into practice. This section provides you with a simple approach based on seven steps. This seven-step model is summarized in Box 10.4 and detailed in the rest of this section.

**Table 10.1** Frameworks for implementing research into practice (from le May 2012)

| Promoting Action on Research Implementation in Health Services (PARiHS) framework (Rycroft-Malone 2010) | Ottawa Model of Research Use (OMRU) (Logan and Graham 2010) | Knowledge-to-Action (KTA) framework (Graham and Tetroe 2010) | Joanna Briggs Institute (JBI) framework for implementing evidence (Pearson 2010) |
|---|---|---|---|
| This framework emphasizes that the success of implementation depends on the relationship between key factors: | This model specifically focuses on getting valid research findings implemented. | This framework is conceptually robust, being derived from an analysis of 31 planned action/change theories in health and social sciences, education and management. | This framework is particularly focused on the use of research evidence. |
| • The nature of the evidence (whether it is research, clinical experience or patient experience) | There are six key structural elements: | The framework emphasizes the importance of social interaction and of tailoring evidence to meet contextual and cultural needs. | At its core there are four key components: • Healthcare evidence generation • Evidence synthesis |
| | 1. The research-informed innovation 2. The potential adopters 3. The practice environment | | • Evidence/knowledge transfer • Evidence utilization |
| • The context within which it is implemented (including the culture of the organization, leadership and the potential for evaluation) | 4. Implementation interventions for transferring the research findings into practice 5. The adoption of the innovation 6. The outcomes – health-related and others | The framework comprises a number of phases: • Identify problem/ select knowledge | Our primary concern is the use of evidence – this part of the framework focuses on practice change, embedding evidence through system/ organization-wide change and evaluating its impact. |
| • The facilitation of this implementation (which depends on the role of the facilitator and their attributes and skills) | In addition there are three process elements that need to be considered (AME): | • Adapt knowledge to the local context • Assess barriers to knowledge use | The framework emphasizes that the process of evidence utilization is influenced by: |
| Successful implementation will occur 'when evidence is scientifically robust and matches professional consensus and patients' preferences … the context receptive to change with sympathetic cultures, strong leadership, and appropriate monitoring and feedback systems … and, when there is | • Assessment of barriers and supports (these are associated with the structural elements 1–3 above) • Monitoring how the research-informed innovation is implemented | • Implement tailored intervention • Monitor knowledge use | • resources; • education/expertise; |

continued ➤

**Table 10.1**  Frameworks for implementing research into practice (from le May 2012)

| Promoting Action on Research Implementation in Health Services (PARiHS) framework (Rycroft-Malone 2010) | Ottawa Model of Research Use (OMRU) (Logan and Graham 2010) | Knowledge-to-Action (KTA) framework (Graham and Tetroe 2010) | Joanna Briggs Institute (JBI) framework for implementing evidence (Pearson 2010) |
|---|---|---|---|
| appropriate facilitation of change with input from skilled external and internal facilitators' (pp 112–113).<br><br>This framework may be used to diagnose the receptiveness of each context to change and thereby tailor any facilitation to meet the needs of that specific context. | • Evaluation of the impact of the innovation (monitoring and evaluation are linked closely to structural elements 4–6)<br><br>This model can be applied to evidence-based practice projects and also quality improvement projects. | • Evaluate outcomes (both those associated with the process of change and the outcomes in relation to healthcare)<br><br>• Sustain knowledge use | • patient preference;<br><br>• the availability of research;<br><br>• staffing levels, skill mix; and<br><br>• policies. |

| Box 10.4 | A simple process to help you to implement research in practice (le May 2001) |
| --- | --- |

1. Identifying areas of care that could be improved by using research.

2. Finding relevant research through searching the literature and asking experts.

3. Assessing the quality of that research.

4. Determining which research provides the best approach to care, is clinically relevant for the patient/service user and can be provided by the organization in which care is being given.

5. Making required changes to practice to incorporate the research findings.

6. Evaluating the impact of that research on the care being provided.

7. Keeping up to date and changing practice accordingly.

## Identifying areas of care that could be improved by using research

In Chapter 5 we started to think about identifying worthwhile questions to answer through research and in Chapter 6 how to assess the quality of various types of research and their clinical relevance. In this chapter we're going to use some of these ideas to consider how to improve care by implementing relevant research. The first step in this process is to identify aspects of care that could be improved upon.

| Box 10.5 | Identifying aspects of care that could be improved if relevant research was implemented |
| --- | --- |

You may be able to identify aspects of care that could be altered through:

- reflecting on your own experience: think about times when you have not known the best way to practise when caring for a patient or when you have found that routine practice does not work for a group of patients;

- considering mistakes, complaints or poor practice that you have heard about: these may have led you to examine how things could have been done differently in order to avoid these errors;

- reading audits of practice that suggest that care could be improved: improvement could be linked to using more up-to-date research findings in practice;

- hearing about research-based changes made to care by others and wanting to use these changes in your own practice.

## Finding relevant research through searching the literature and asking experts

Once you've identified an aspect of care that needs to be improved you need to think about searching and appraising the literature to see what research is available to help you make that improvement. In order to do this you need to list important key words related to the topic you're interested in and then search a variety of databases and internet sites (see Box 10.6), using the key words, to identify relevant papers, systematic reviews of research (collections of appraised studies) and guidelines (most of which are based on sound research evidence). You'll be using the searching skills that you've already learned to help you to find literature for assignments.

In addition to searching databases and internet sites yourself, it's useful to ask a librarian for help and also to ask colleagues, particularly those seen as experts in your chosen area, what they know. Such shortcuts are very helpful, not only saving you time but perhaps also highlighting research that isn't available through conventional database and internet searches.

---

**Box 10.6    Some useful databases**

Cumulative Index of Nursing and Allied Health Literature (CINAHL) (**www.ebscohost.com/cinahl**)

MEDLINE (**www.nlm.nih.gov**)

NHS Evidence (**www.evidence.nhs.uk/nhs-evidence-content/journals-and-databases**)

The Cochrane Library (**www.thecochranelibrary.com/view/0/index.html**) incorporating:

- the Cochrane Database of Systematic Reviews (CDSR)
- the Database of Abstracts of Reviews of Effectiveness (DARE)
- the Cochrane Controlled Trials Register (CCTR)
- the Cochrane Review Methodology Database

The National Institute for Health and Clinical Excellence (NICE) (for guidelines) (**www.nice. org.uk/guidance/index.jsp?action=byType&type=2&status=3**)

Google Scholar (**http://scholar.google.co.uk/**)

You can find unpublished literature using GreyNet (**www.greynet.org/**)

---

Always keep a record of the searches you've made and the results that you came up with. This will help you to locate information again if you need to and also to tell other people how you found your information. Doing this will save you a lot of time.

When you have your list of papers, reviews and guidelines, start to prioritize and reduce them by reading their abstracts/summaries in order to decide which ones really are relevant and which aren't. Titles by themselves can be very misleading: sometimes a title can make you think that the work is about people like the patients you are caring for, but when you read further, you find it is not. As soon as you have your prioritized list, locate and retrieve the papers so that you can assess which pieces of information are going to be good enough to use in practice.

## Assessing the quality of the selected research

Assessing the quality of any research is about determining how rigorous the process of undertaking that research has been. The first questions you need to pose, to assess the quality of any sort of research paper, are very general ones (see Box 10.7). Once you have answered these questions you can decide whether the research is good enough to move on to the next, more specific, stage of quality assessment. If it is not, simply remove it from your list. (For instance, I would exclude papers with a mismatch between the research question and the findings presented or where the design and methods for data collection and analysis were not clearly stated and were confusing.)

When you're thinking about systematic reviews of research, use the checklist devised by the Critical Appraisal Skills Programme (CASP) to guide you – you can find this at **www.sph.nhs.uk/sph-files/casp-appraisal-tools/S.Reviews%20Appraisal%20Tool.pdf/view.**

| Box 10.7 | General questions to ask about research papers (adapted from De Poy and Gitlin 1994) |
|---|---|

- Was the study clear?
- Was the research question clearly stated?
- What was the purpose?
- Did the research design and methods fit the purpose?
- Was the literature review relevant?
- Was the literature review systematic?
- Were threats to reliability and validity acknowledged? And controlled?
- Were issues related to the credibility of the research considered?
- Was the analysis clear?
- Do the findings address the research question?
- Are the implications for practice acknowledged?
- Do the conclusions fit with the data presented?
- Are ethical considerations discussed?
- Who undertook the research?
- Who funded the work?
- Do you have enough information to repeat the study?

After you've done this preliminary filtering, sort the remaining studies by design and read them critically again with the criteria for evaluation of specific research designs in mind (see Chapter 6). You will also find it helpful to use the specific CASP tools recommended above now. Use the same filtering process – if the study is good enough, keep it; if not, disregard it. This stage will help you to further reduce your list until you have only the key studies, of good quality, left to base your practice on.

## Determining whether research will be clinically relevant to patients/service users

Using your now shortened list of studies, decide which ones are actually relevant to the patients with whom you are working. This is a very important step since some research, even that of high quality, will be useful only to a very few patients/service users, or will be too expensive to implement within the budgets of your unit/organization, or simply impracticable to implement in the time available to you. It is therefore vital to make this assessment before implementing research into practice. Box 10.8 gives you a number of useful questions to answer in order to guide your decision making.

| Box 10.8 | Establishing clinical relevance – useful questions to ask (le May 1999; le May and Gabbay 2011) |
|---|---|

Is the evidence relevant clinically for the patient/service user?

1. Could this research be used in my practice arena? (If not, why not?)

2. What benefits will the implementation of this evidence have for patients/carers/staff?

3. What risks are associated with implementation/non-implementation?

Can the evidence be used by the organization within which care is being given?

1. Are there enough resources for implementation?

2. What are the opportunities for and constraints on implementing this evidence?

Remember to talk to other people and ask their opinions as well. Some of these questions might be difficult for you to answer by yourself.

## Making required changes to practice to incorporate the research findings

Once you've decided to implement any research findings you will need to think about how to change practice. There are many techniques that you can use. You can find out more about these by going to the National Institute for Health Research Service Delivery and Organisation programme website (www.sdo.nihr.ac.uk) and looking at the reports under the section called 'Managing change in the NHS' found under 'Publications' in 'News, publications and events'. The most useful one is *Organisational Change* (Iles and Sutherland 2001), which details all the main approaches to change management. You can download it at www.sdo.nihr.ac.uk/files/adhoc/change-management-review.pdf. You will need to select an approach that best fits the context in which you're working and your own skills.

It is important to remember that, in order to implement any change, you need to persuade other people that the change will be worthwhile, so you need to think about why you think changes should be made. Here are some reasons why nurses think that changing practice is worthwhile:

1. To make practice more effective
2. To make practice more cost-effective
3. To make practice of better quality
4. To make practice more accessible and equitable
5. To make practice more appropriate
6. To make practice better matched to service users' expectations
7. To make practice more satisfying – for the nurse and for the service user

Jot down any other general reasons that you can think of. You will need to make these more specific to your patient group and the findings that you intend to implement in order to make your arguments more relevant and convincing.

## Evaluating the impact on care of research that you have used

An essential last step in this process is to make an assessment of how the research that you've implemented has impacted on the care that you provide. This can very simply be done by noting in your care plan what you have done and how this has benefited (or not) the patient. It should become part of your daily routine assessment/evaluation of care and needs to be communicated to your colleagues. Although longer-term evaluations are important (see Chapter 11), undertaking these is probably beyond your scope of practice at the moment.

## Keeping up to date and changing practice accordingly

This final component will be relevant to you throughout your career since keeping your knowledge and skills updated is an essential facet of being a nurse. Eventually you will find that many sorts of knowledge – from, for example, your readings of research, theory, audit and policy – are melded together with your experiences to form what people are beginning to refer to as 'mindlines' (Gabbay and le May 2011). Researchers have found that mindlines guide your practice. Mindlines are:

> ... internalized, collectively reinforced and often tacit guidelines that are informed by clinicians' training, by their own and each other's experience, by their interactions with their role sets, by their reading, by the way they have learnt to handle the [ir] conflicting demands, by their understanding of local circumstances and systems, and by a host of other sources ... Clinicians build up mindlines as a bank of personalized, flexible syntheses of all the different types of theoretical and experiential knowledge that they need to be able to call upon instantaneously.
>
> (Gabbay and le May 2011 pp 43–44)

You will develop a collection of mindlines as you become more established in your profession. Eventually you will find that this collection not only gives you the confidence to practise competently but also enables you to articulate evidence that can be used to persuade others to change their practice and integrate relevant research findings into practice.

# ■ References

Cooksey D. A Review of UK Health Research funding. HM Treasury 2006. Available at: **www.hm-treasury.gov.uk/cooksey_review_index.htm.** Accessed 19 February 2012.

Cullum N, Cilisha D, Maynes B, Marks S. *Evidence-based Nursing: An introduction.* 2008; Oxford: Blackwell.

De Poy E, Gitlin L. *Introduction to Research. Understanding and Applying Multiple Strategies.* 1994; St Louis, MO: Mosby.

Gabbay J, le May A. *Practice Based Evidence for Healthcare: Clinical mindlines.* 2011; London: Routledge.

Gerrish K, Ashworth P, Lacey A, Bailey J. Developing evidence-based practice: experiences of senior and junior clinical nurses. *Journal of Advanced Nursing.* 2008; **62**(1): 62–73.

Graham I, Tetroe J. The knowledge to action framework. In: J Rycroft-Malone, T Bucknall (eds). *Models and Frameworks for Implementing Evidence-Based Practice: Linking evidence to action.* 2010; Oxford: Wiley-Blackwell.

Iles I, Sutherland S. *Organisational Change.* 2001; London: National Co-ordinating Centre for NHS Service Delivery and Organisation R & D.

Kajermo K, Boström A-M, Thompson D, Hutchinson A, Estabrooks C, Wallin L. The BARRIERS scale – the barriers to research utilization scale: a systematic review. *Implementation Science.* 2010; **5**: 32.

Kitson AL, Harvey G, McCormack B. Enabling the implementation of evidence based practice: a conceptual framework. *Quality in Health Care.* 1998; **7**: 149–158.

le May A. Evidence based practice. *Nursing Times Clinical Monograph No 1.* 1999; London: EMAP.

le May A. *Making Use of Research.* 2001; London: South Bank University, Distance Learning Centre.

le May A. Developing expert practice. In: D Barton, A le May (eds). *Adult Nursing: Preparing for practice.* 2012; London: Hodder Arnold.

le May A, Gabbay J. Evidence based practice in practice. In: G Lewith, J Cousins, H Walach (eds). *Clinical Research in Complementary Therapies.* 2011; Edinburgh: Elsevier.

le May A, Mulhall A, Alexander C. Bridging the research–practice gap: exploring the research cultures of practitioners and managers. *Journal of Advanced Nursing.* 1998; **28**(2): 428–437.

Logan J, Graham I. The Ottawa Model of Research Use. In: J Rycroft-Malone, T Bucknall (eds). *Models and Frameworks for Implementing Evidence-Based Practice: Linking evidence to action.* 2010; Oxford: Wiley-Blackwell.

Pearson A. The Joanna Briggs Institute model of evidence-based health care as a framework for implementing evidence. In: J Rycroft-Malone, T Bucknall (eds). *Models and Frameworks for Implementing Evidence-Based Practice: Linking evidence to action.* 2010; Oxford: Wiley-Blackwell.

Profetto-McGrath J, Smith K, Hugo K, Taylor M, El-Hajj H. Clinical nurse specialists' use of evidence in practice: a pilot study. *Worldviews on Evidence-Based Nursing.* 2007; **4**(2): 86–96.

Rycroft-Malone J. Promoting Action on Research Implementation in Health Services (PARiHS). In: J Rycroft-Malone, T Bucknall (eds). *Models and Frameworks for Implementing Evidence-Based Practice: Linking evidence to action.* 2010; Oxford: Wiley-Blackwell.

Thompson D, Estabrooks C, Scott-Findlay S, Moore K, Wallin L. Interventions aimed at increasing research use in nursing: a systematic review. *Implementation Science.* 2007; **2**:15.

United Kingdom Clinical Research Collaboration. Developing the best research professionals. Qualified graduate nurses: recommendations for preparing and supporting clinical academic nurses of the future. 2007; Report of the UKCRC Subcommittee for Nurses in Clinical Research (Workforce). London: UKCRC.

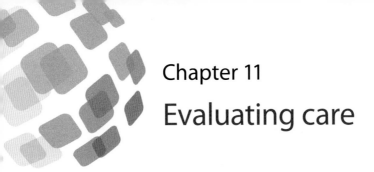

# Chapter 11

# Evaluating care

## ▪ Introduction

This chapter focuses on some of the ways through which nurses can evaluate care, systematically and rigorously, without doing research. Developing an evaluative approach to providing care is very important if you're going to deliver clinically effective care for your patients/service users. The chapter starts by considering what clinical effectiveness is and then moves on to describe how you might achieve this by using clinical audit, quality improvement techniques and evaluative reflective practice.

## ▪ Clinical effectiveness

Clinical effectiveness is about providing the best possible healthcare to people with the resources available. In 1996 the Department of Health defined clinical effectiveness as:

*the extent to which specific clinical interventions when deployed in the field for a particular patient or population do what they are intended to do, i.e. maintain and improve health and secure the greatest possible health gain from the available resources.*

That same year, the RCN described clinical effectiveness as building on audit and quality improvement in order to provide a 'framework for linking research, implementation and evaluation in clinical practice' (p3). This framework has more recently been portrayed, at a more personal level, by NHS Quality Improvement Scotland (NHS QIS 2005) as:

- *the right person (you) doing;*
- *the right thing (evidence based practice);*

- *in the right way (skills and competence);*
- *at the right time (providing treatment/services when the patient needs them);*
- *in the right place (location of treatment/services);*
- *with the right result (clinical effectiveness/maximising health gain).*

(www.clinicalgovernance.scot.nhs.uk/section2/definition.asp)

In order to do this:

- *We need to have information available* not only about the care that is being delivered – its effectiveness and efficiency – but also any new research evidence about the best care to provide and the best ways through which care could be delivered.
- *We need to openly scrutinize the delivery of care.* Practitioners, managers and support workers always need to be thinking about what they do and how they could do things better or more safely. This process needs to be logical and reviewed by others within the team providing health (and social) care. It is the opposite to practising traditionally or ritualistically – a criticism that is made of some nurses.
- *We should include people who use healthcare services* in this process. Service users are key drivers for clinical effectiveness and it's important to try wherever possible to co-design services with them (Bates and Robert 2006). The Picker Institute Europe published a set of principles related to patient-centred care which should be kept in mind when anyone is thinking about clinical effectiveness. They focus on:
  - respect for patients' values, preference and expressed needs;
  - coordination and integration of care;
  - information, communication and education;
  - physical comfort;
  - emotional support and alleviation of fear and anxiety;
  - involvement of family and friends;
  - continuity and transition;
  - access to care.

  If you go to the website (**http://pickerinstitute.org/about/picker-principles/**) you will find more information about each of these principles and a series of short video clips.
- *We need to identify where change is needed* and ensure that that change is based on evidence from research, examples of best practice from elsewhere or audit. Change should be managed in a purposeful way to make its implementation as effective and efficient as possible.
- *We should ensure that all change is evaluated* to determine the extent of its success and altered if need be.
- *We must tell others about what has been done* through either publications or formal/informal presentations. Failure to do this may be why information about the best care often fails to get across to everyone who needs to know and care in some areas stagnates.

This process needs to be carried out by everyone. Clinical effectiveness is not just the concern of those providing direct patient care, it needs to be the concern of their managers and their managers, too. In other words, clinical effectiveness needs to be a concern of everyone in every organization (or group of organizations) who provides health and social care.

In order to know that our care is clinically effective, we need to know what the outcomes of our care are and how these could be improved. This is where audit, quality improvement techniques and evaluative reflective practice fit in.

## ■ Clinical audit

The Healthcare Quality Improvement Partnership (HQIP) (**www.hqip.org.uk**) was created in 2008 to promote quality in healthcare and increase the impact of clinical audit. Clinical audit is:

> *A quality improvement process that seeks to improve patient care and outcomes through systematic review of care against explicit criteria and the implementation of change. Put more simply: clinical audit is all about measuring the quality of care and services against agreed standards and making improvements where necessary.*
> (*NHS Clinical Governance Support Team 2002*)

Audit is always a cyclical process which is about measuring care against agreed criteria (or standards), deciding whether alterations need to be made to care, making changes, and measuring again to see whether the change has been effective (see Figure 11.1).

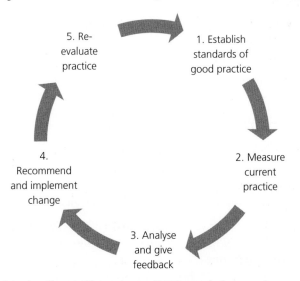

**Figure 11.1** The clinical audit cycle (Kongnyuy *et al* 2008: **www.rrh.org.au**)

Audit can be done either at national or at local level. You are likely to have come across both types of audit in your readings, but you are more likely to be involved in local audit. Copeland (2005) has laid out a set of criteria that you might find useful either when taking part in audit or later, when designing audit yourself (see Box 11.1).

| Box 11.1 | The top dozen: criteria for 'good local clinical audit' (Copeland 2005 p16) |
|---|---|

1.  Should be part of a structured programme.
2.  Topics chosen should in the main be high risk, high volume or high cost or reflect National Clinical Audits, NSFs (National Service Frameworks) or NICE guidance.
3.  Service users should be part of the clinical audit process.
4.  Should be multidisciplinary in nature.
5.  Clinical audit should include assessment of process and outcome of care.
6.  Standards should be derived from good quality guidelines.
7.  The sample size chosen should be adequate to produce credible results.
8.  Managers should be actively involved in audit and in particular in the development of action plans from audit enquiry.
9.  Action plans should address the local barriers to change and identify those responsible for service improvement.
10. Re-audit should be applied to ascertain whether improvements in care have been implemented as a result of clinical audit.
11. Systems, structures and specific mechanisms should be made available to monitor service improvements once the audit cycle has been completed.
12. Each audit should have a local lead.

Doing audit is not the same as doing research or service evaluation, but people often confuse them. In order to minimize this confusion, the National Research Ethics Service (NRES) (2007) formulated Table 11.1 and it is included here to help you distinguish between these three important facets of evaluative practice.

## ■ Quality improvement techniques

Quality improvement (QI) is

> *a formal approach to the analysis of performance and systematic efforts to improve it ... QI involves both prospective and retrospective reviews. It is aimed at improvement – measuring where you are, and figuring out ways to make things better. It specifically attempts to avoid attributing blame, and to create systems to prevent errors from happening.*
>
> *(Duke University 2005)* (http://patientsafetyed.duhs.duke.edu/module_a/ introduction/introduction.html).

**Table 11.1** The differences between audit, research and service evaluation (NRES 2007) (**www.red.mmu.ac.uk/documents/res_files/ethics/NRES_leaflet_Defining_Research-1.pdf**)

| Research | Clinical audit | Service evaluation |
| --- | --- | --- |
| The attempt to derive generalisable new knowledge including studies that aim to generate hypotheses, as well as studies that aim to test them. | Designed and conducted to produce information to inform delivery of best care. | Designed and conducted solely to define or judge current care. |
| Quantitative research – designed to test a hypothesis. Qualitative research – identifies/ explores themes following established methodology. | Designed to answer the question: 'Does this service reach a predetermined standard?' | Designed to answer the question: 'What standard does this service achieve?' |
| Addresses clearly defined questions, aims and objectives. | Measures against a standard. | Measures current service without reference to a standard. |
| Quantitative research – may involve evaluating or comparing interventions, particularly new ones. Qualitative research – usually involves studying how interventions and relationships are experienced. | Involves an intervention in use only (the choice of treatment is that of the clinician and patient according to guidance, professional standards and/or patient preference). | Involves an intervention in use only (the choice of treatment is that of the clinician and patient according to guidance, professional standards and/or patient preference). |
| Usually involves collecting data that are additional to those for routine care but may include data collected routinely. May involve treatments, samples or investigations additional to routine care. | Usually involves analysis of existing data, but may include administration of simple interview or questionnaire. | Usually involves analysis of existing data, but may include administration of simple interview or questionnaire. |
| Quantitative research – study design may involve allocating patients to intervention groups. Qualitative research uses a clearly defined sampling framework underpinned by conceptual or theoretical justifications. | No allocation to intervention groups: the healthcare professional and patient have chosen intervention before clinical audit. | No allocation to intervention groups: the healthcare professional and patient have chosen intervention before service evaluation. |
| May involve randomisation. | No randomisation. | No randomisation. |

Some examples of quality improvement techniques that you may be familiar with include the Deming Cycle (better known as the Plan, Do, Study, Act (PDSA) cycle) and LEAN thinking. Originally developed from the car-making industry they are now being successfully used in healthcare settings across the world to analyse and improve the process of care delivery and its outcome for patients (and staff). Despite using different methods (see Box 11.2 and page 141), they essentially aim to do one thing: help us to determine whether the care given to patients is as good as it possibly could be and if not they provide us with ways to identify how care could be improved.

---

### Exercise 11.1  Thinking about quality improvement

Identify an area of your current practice that you think should be improved. Jot down some thoughts in relation to the following questions:

What precisely needs to be improved?

Why?

Who agrees with you that improvement is needed?

Who disagrees with you?

Read more about quality improvement techniques starting with the information in Box 11.1. Then think about the following questions in relation to your area for improvement:

What do you propose to do in order to make this improvement?

Would a quality improvement technique help you in this process? If so, which one and why?

---

| Box 11.2 | Summary of the PDSA cycle |
|---|---|

The PDSA cycle, popularized by the Institute for Healthcare Improvement (IHI) (**www.ihi.org/ IHI/**) in North America, has been used across the world in order to make improvements to healthcare. Essentially it is about finding the answers to three key questions:

What are we trying to accomplish?

What change can we make that will result in an improvement?

How will we know that a change is an improvement?

The cycle is used for 'testing a change by developing a plan to test the change (Plan), carrying out the test (Do), observing and learning from the consequences (Study) and determining what modifications should be made to the test (Act)' (**www.ihi.org/IHI/Topics/ Improvement/ImprovementMethods/Tools/ Plan-Do-Study-Act%20(PDSA)%20 Worksheet**).

---

The PDSA cycle is most often associated with small-scale change at particular hot spots in an organization or a particular care pathway. Although we often read about PDSA being used by healthcare workers, it can be effectively used by volunteers or lay carers. Maurice Wilson (2005), a volunteer with the Healthy Communities Collaborative in

Northampton, writes about what it was like to use the PDSA cycle to help change services within his local community. The collaborative used the PDSA cycle to place the onus for action on the community volunteers and, by doing this, enabled them 'to work in equal partnership with health professions. The beauty of the project was that it was "action-based", which meant success rested with community volunteers themselves: it was about people feeling included in any change and their contributions and opinions being valued' (Wilson 2005 p127).

LEAN thinking is often described as a way of achieving larger-scale change across an organization(s) and takes a somewhat different approach to the PDSA cycle. Refined by Toyota, this approach has been adapted for use in healthcare (see Miller 2005 and DH 2008), but probably the best known use of LEAN thinking in nursing is the work undertaken on the 'Productive Ward' initiative supported by the Institute for Innovation and Improvement from 2007. LEAN thinking (**www.lean.org/**) essentially seeks to do more with less, the emphasis being to strip out waste from the system (e.g. waste of money, resources, time and good will) so that care can be provided, to the highest possible standard, in the most cost-effective way. Various techniques are used within the LEAN thinking process (for a useful summary go to **www.atoshealthcare.com/ UserFiles/File/fact-sheets/2642-0609%20Achieving%20Lean%20and%20healthy%20 transformation%20FS.pdf**).

Sometimes LEAN thinking is linked to Six Sigma, a very quantitative approach. Six Sigma has five phases: define, measure, analyse, improve and control (DMAIC). The first phase includes a cost–benefit analysis and only if this is acceptable should the project progress any further. In the measurement phase, baseline data are collected to help the project team understand and quantify what is happening at the outset. This information can then be used to design a solution which will improve care and produce measurable outcomes that will show success at subsequent monitoring. For more information go to **www.isixsigma.com**.

## ■ Evaluative reflective practice

Evaluative reflective practice is about critically reviewing the care that you have given in order to identify if (and how) you could do it differently (i.e. better) the next time. Whether you do this with colleagues or on your own, you will find it useful to have a structure to guide your reflection. The best approach, and one that you may have come across already, is Gibbs' (1988) reflective cycle (see Figure 11.2).

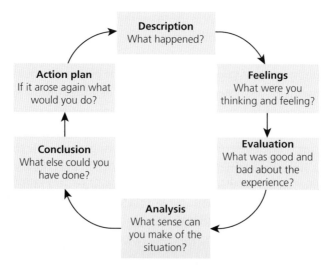

**Figure 11.2** Gibbs' reflective cycle (**http://jolt.merlot.org/vol7no1/images/park_fig2.jpg**)

Clinical audit, quality improvement techniques and evaluative reflective practice are all structured, systematic ways of determining the effectiveness of practice. Although each approach is structured differently, they all have at their core three unifying characteristics. First, the goal of improving care; second, a systematic approach to assessing what has been done and what needs to be done; and third, the requirement to change practice in order to make it better (this change should have a rigorous evidence base).

## Measuring care

Let's now turn our attention to measuring these changes. In order to determine whether care is improving, whether through clinical audit, quality improvement or evaluative reflective practice, we need to be able to measure care. Measurement of nursing care has recently become an important area of concern, with the Royal College of Nursing publishing a position statement in relation to its importance (RCN 2009). You can access this statement at **www.rcn.org.uk/__data/assets/pdf_file/0004/248872/003535.pdf**.

In this statement, the RCN puts forward a number of tenets on quality measurement. The last one is of the most use when we think about measuring care. It simply states that 'good indicators are those suited to their intended purpose, are relevant, valid, reliable, feasible and useful in supporting change' (p5). When you're thinking about how to measure your improvements you need to have these in your mind to ensure that the measures you use to evaluate care are:

- suited to their intended purpose;
- relevant;

- valid;
- reliable;
- feasible (to use);
- useful in supporting change.

# Conclusions

Making care more effective means that everyone involved in providing care should take responsibility for its delivery, alteration and evaluation. This process needs to blend the systematic study of the process of care with evidence-based decision making. While a range of techniques is available to guide this process, undertaking it will also rely on the knowledge and skills that you have and the people you work with.

# Further reading

Read about how the Productive Ward scheme is progressing in: The Productive Ward: What do we know about uptake and impact on staff and patients? *Policy+*. 2010; **24** (www.kcl. ac.uk/content/1/c6/06/89/90/PolicyIssue24.pdf).

Look at: Can you measure nursing? *Policy+*. 2008; **12** to see what nurse researchers think about measuring nursing (www.kcl.ac.uk/content/1/c6/04/37/70/PolicyIssue12.pdf).

# References

Bates P, Robert G. Experience-based design: from redesigning the system around the patient to co-designing services with the patient. *Quality and Safety in Health Care*. 2006; **15**: 307–310.

Copeland G. *A Practical Handbook for Clinical Audit*. 2005; NHS Clinical Governance Support Team. Available at: www.wales.nhs.uk/sites3/Documents/501/Practical_Clinical_Audit_Handbook_v1_1.pdf. Accessed 22 October 2011.

Department of Health. *Promoting Clinical Effectiveness: A framework for action in and through the NHS*. 1996; London: NHS Executive.

Department of Health. *High Quality Care for All. NHS Next Stage Review Final Report*. 2008; London: DH.

Duke University. *Patient Safety – Quality Improvement*. 2005. Available at: http://patientsafetyed.duhs.duke.edu/. Accessed 22 October 2011.

Gibbs G. *Learning by Doing: A guide to teaching and learning methods*. 1988; Oxford: Further Education Unit, Oxford Polytechnic.

Kongnyuy EJ, Mlava G, van den Broek N. Establishing standards for obstructed labour in a low-income country. *Rural and Remote Health*. 2008; **8**: (1022).

Miller D. *Going Lean in Health Care*. 2005; Cambridge, MA: Institute for Healthcare Improvement.

National Research Ethics Service. *Defining Research*. 2007. Available at: **www.red.mmu. ac.uk/documents/res_files/ethics/NRES_leaflet_Defining_Research-1.pdf**. Accessed 22 October 2011.

NHS Clinical Governance Support Team. 2002; accessed via Health Quality Improvement Partnership (**www.hqip.org.uk**).

NHS QIS. 2005. Available at: **www.clinicalgovernance.scot.nhs.uk/section2/definition.asp**. Accessed 16 October 2010.

RCN. *Measuring for Quality in Health and Social Care. An RCN position statement*. 2009; London: Royal College of Nursing.

Wilson M. Preventing falls in older people. In: M Rawlins, P Littlejohns (eds). *Delivering Quality in the NHS*. 2005; Oxford: Radcliffe.

# Index

Abbreviations used: EBP, evidence-based practice; QL, quality of life.